SPASM

SPASM:

Why Your Body
is Painfully Tight
and How You Can Loosen it . . .
for Good!

by JOHN C. LOWE, M.A., D.C.
Foreword by Robert S. Mendelsohn, M.D.
Cover and illustrations by Jan Zollars

McDOWELL PUBLISHING COMPANY / HOUSTON, TEXAS

Library of Congress Catalog Card Co. 83-62566

ISBN—Soft: 0-914609-00-9   15.00

McDowell Publishing Company

POBox 980005   Houston, Texas 77098

To my mother, Evelyn E. Lowe, for
her love, dedication, and support
through my decade of formal education
and through my subsequent years of
real education.

CONTENTS

FOREWORD

I knew nothing about chiropractors until I entered medical school where I was taught never to "consort" (that was the exact word that was used) with chiropractors. Some years later I was allowed to associate with them. Early in the '80s I participated in legal action brought by the chiropractors against the American Medical Association. As a result of that lawsuit, I am now permitted to consult with chiropractors. And, before too many years pass, I predict MDs will be free to marry chiropractors.

Like all other medical students, I was taught the standard answers to patients who reported they had been cured at the hands of chiropractors. These responses included "You're lucky"—or the ever-popular "Spontaneous remission." Indeed, to this day I am frustrated at the ability of chiropractors to achieve "spontaneous remission" in patients with heart disease, arthritis, cancer and other serious chronic ailments. It seems that we MDs do not get our fair share. Why must I advise patients: If you want a spontaneous remission, see a chiropractor.

In the mid-70s, I served as a member, and later chairman, of the State of Illinois Medical Licensure Board. A combined Board, it included five MDs, one osteopath and one chiropractor. I have always wondered why one chiropractor was worth five MDs!

While testifying in one of my frequent court appearances on behalf of chiropractors, the opposing lawyer challenged me on cross-examination, "Doctor, do you know anything about the theory of chiropractic?" Aware of the pitfall of a negative answer, I promptly and energetically responded, "Oh, yes. I know all about the theory of chiropractic." Moving in for the kill, the attorney not unexpectedly requested, "Please tell us what you know." With all the innocence I could muster, I said, "My wife's back trouble was cured by a chiropractor after three orthopedic specialists had failed."

"Dr. Mendelsohn," he said condescendingly, "that isn't theory, that's pragmatism." I answered, "Well, pragmatism is my theory." He shot back, "Doctor, you're engaging in tautology." I begged off with, "Despite my university degrees, I'm just a small-town country doctor from Chicago. Would you explain to me what 'tautology' means?"

These and many other happy encounters with chiropractic—the bete noire of Modern Medicine—motivated me to listen closely to those chiropractors to whom, for many years, I have been referring patients (and they have reciprocated). In addition, I have had splendid opportunities to exchange views with chiropractors whom I have met at their organizations' meetings. I watched chiropractic students whom I met as a result of invitations to speak at their colleges. And I read articles and books by chiropractors—in this country and internationally. In my academic position at the University of Illinois College of Medicine as Associate Professor of Preventive Medicine and Community Health, I counselled my medical students to particularly study the New Zealand Report on Chiropractic. Since finishing my 24 year career on the faculties of both Northwestern Medical School and the University of Illinois, I have continued to advise medical students (most recently as Keynote Speaker at the 1983 Annual Convention of the American Medical Students' Association) to make friends with a chiropractor. I have taught that no patient with back trouble should have surgery or drugs without prior approval by a chiropractor. (Similarly, no woman in labor should have a Caesarian section without prior approval by a midwife, and no heart patients should have by-pass surgery without prior approval by a nutritionist.)

Now, Dr. John Lowe has written a book that I will unreservedly recommend to medical students with the assurance that they will seldom face a patient who cannot benefit from Dr. Lowe's wisdom.

However, very few medical students will be able to heed my advice to read this book. Aside from memorizing their origins and insertions, medical students learn almost nothing about muscles, and even less about fascia. They learn nothing about nutrition since Modern Medicine believes not in nutrition, but in "better living through chemistry." They learn precious little about pharmacology, formal training in this vital discipline occupying an average of 60 hours during four years of medical school. Training in medical specialties where they might be able to find out about muscles and myofascial spasm—such as Physical Medicine and Rehabilitation —is optional—not required—in medical school.

But don't think that doctors learn nothing in medical school. They may not learn how to effectively heal. But they do learn how to hate. They learn to despise, denigrate, derogate, detest, and if possible, destroy the enemies of the Religion of Modern Medicine—chiropractic and naprapathy included.

The few who escape the powerful brain-washing of medical education may read and learn from Dr. Lowe. But there is little point in limiting to medical students my recommendation to read *Spasm*.

This is a book for all people—for patients with all kinds of illnesses, for those who have heard the dreary catechism taught to medical novitiates in the seminaries they call medical schools and automatically intoned by doctor-priests— "It's all in your head," "You'll have to learn to live with it," "Just take these pills and trust me."

But Dr. Lowe's book is not just for patients. His clarity of expression, thorough documentation, and ability to cut through complicated subject matter make this a valuable book for relatives and friends of patients. His theoretical interpretations and practical instructions make *Spasm* required reading for athletes, athletic instructors and coaches.

For healthy people—with or without professional education—who possess intellectual curiosity, *Spasm* is the most thoughtful, rational, stimulating approach to muscles I have seen. *Spasm* makes muscles exciting! It represents the definitive statement today on the function and malfunction of muscles and fascia.

Dr. John Lowe's *Spasm* constitutes powerful evidence that chiropractic/naprapathy is fully prepared to fill the vacuum left by the bankruptcy of Modern Medicine. The enthusiastic public reception that I predict his work will receive will signify that chiropractic is now part of mainstream America.

> —Robert S. Mendelsohn, M.D.
> Author, *Confessions of a Medical Heretic*
> September, 1983

ACKNOWLEDGMENTS

I wish to thank:

- Dorinda Bain, Brian Bain, and Dr. Jennifer F. Zea for their help in preparing the manuscript;

- Linda Dozoretz, Judy Moson, and Stephanie Martin for the comforting and reassuring manner in which they've counselled me, and Joel Parker for making it fun; and

- A kind and generous man whose name I can't mention, lest he be punished for his expert help.

A LETTER
TO HEALING ARTS
PRACTITIONERS

January 15, 1983

Re: *"Functionally-induced myofascopathy"*

Dear Practitioner:

    The subject of this book has been speculated about and investigated for at least 140 years. The clinical phenomenon has been variously termed fibrositis, interstitial myofibrositis, muscle calluses, muscle gelling or myogeloses, myalgic spots, trigger points, muscle hardenings, muscular rheumatism, non-articular rheumatism, soft-part rheumatism, myofascial pain syndrome, myofascitis, as well as other names and phrases. I feel that all these names, if they're intended to represent the phenomenon I discuss in this book, are inadequate in at least one respect: they don't comprehensively describe the *process* involved. This process appears to follow what we know to be the body's characteristic response to irritation. The process begins as a functional adaptation and, as it continues beyond its usefulness, ends as a pathological conversion of muscle and fascia to almost lifeless fibrous adhesions. I believe, ergo, that a preferable designation for the process is the more comprehensive term, "functionally-induced myofascopathy."

I agree with others who have reviewed the literature on this phenomenon: The data available to date lead to few exactitudes regarding the etiology and nature of the lesions involved. I believe, though, that the inconsistency of the research findings is based upon the tremendous anatomical, physiological, and biochemical variability of human beings, and consequently, their variable reactions to the same or similar stresses.

I also believe that as more data accumulate, these will etch more clearly the pattern that to me already seems hazily obvious. That pattern is this: Persistent mechanical, biochemical and psychological stresses induce hypermyotonia; this torques and compresses the fascial tissues in which free nerve endings (which mediate pain) are embedded and through which vascular and neural pathways course to nourish and innervate muscles; chronic obstruction of the vascular pathways and irritation of the neural receptors disrupt the normal chemistry and physiology of the muscles and fascia, and inflammation and/or deterioration ensue; the end lesion is a deteriorative product that exhibits the characteristics of fibrous adhesions; and as these contract (a process called physiological creep) the end attachments of the involved myofascial tissues are approximated, distorting structure, limiting flexibility, further obstructing vascular channels, and exciting nociceptors; and these pathogenic sequelae to some extent impede normal biochemical and physiological processes anatomically remote from the central myofascopathic locus.

I believe the three stages of this process as I've described it —adaptation, inflammation, and deterioration—while oversimplified, are accurate. This, however, is of only secondary importance to me; for whether or not this working hypothesis is correct, the therapeutic and rehabilitative measures that derive from the hypothesis *are* clinically effective, and this to me is of *supreme* importance. Hypotheses come and go, but empirically effective treatments persist. I agree with Bonney Prudden in regard to this matter: The treatment works, and it would be inhumane to withhold it from the public until the pathophysiology is concretely elucidated.

I've entitled this book *Spasm,* despite Kraft, Johnson and LaBan's argument that their electromyographic measures demonstrate electrochemical silence in what some clinicians and investigators choose to call "muscle spasms." I've done so for four reasons: 1) On theoretical and experiential grounds, I believe spasms to be a prerequisite to and an integral stage in the process of functionally-induced myofascopathy; 2) the term "spasm," while perhaps not corresponding to acute cramps (such as nocturnal cramps in people with impaired circulation), is for the general public a suitable surrogate for the jargonistic terms *hypermyotonia* and *contracture;* 3) I know that it's at *this* stage of the phenomenon, at the point of spasm, that procedures can most productively be applied to free patients from the process; and 4) both the spinal reflex archs and cortical correlates of the process tend themselves to generate hypermyotonia, so that whether cause, effect, or both, spasms are a concomitant of the process, and mitigating these spasms is critical for patients' wellbeing . . . and after all, it *is* for them that this self-help book is intended.

MEDICAL AND OSTEOPATHIC DOCTORS

At various points throughout this book, I make statements about what I feel to be some dangers of modern allopathic medicine and most of its practitioners. I do so mainly because Modern Medicine seems to be involved in a mobster-like collusion with the pharmaceutical industry. This collusion, as I see it, has resulted in Modern Medicine: 1) foregoing a rational search for harmless and effective health care methods, while steadfastly administering drugs for any and every health problem, even those for which drugs are blatantly inappropriate, such as functional spasms; 2) viciously opposing harmless and efficacious forms of therapy that might seriously compete with the toxic and deadly products of the drug industry; and 3) oppressing and persecuting those who promulgate these alternative forms of treatment. I therefore see modern allopathic medicine and most of its practitioners as the strong-arm of the drug industry, inculcated in the public mind as *the* authorities on health, and given the power to pass deadly judgment on any person or group that dares compete with the drug industry's "market."

I wholeheartedly support a *reasonable* sense of discrimination in health care—that is, encouraging treatments that show promise of helping human beings, while discouraging useless treatments that accomplish little more than exploitation. But political medicine has used the "sense of discrimination" quite *un*reasonably; it has flagrantly misused it as a club to bludgeon whole professions (chiropractic, dentistry, podiatry, optometry, clinical psychology, naturapathy, and naprapathy) that constitute competition to allopathic medicine and its allied industries. As a result, political medicine's abuse of this "sense of discrimination" has inflicted untold suffering on human beings.

Political medicine has smudged the face of even the altruistic, humane allopathic practitioner. As a result, hordes of people have turned to alternative—and unfortunately, in some cases, worthless—methods in the pursuit of health. I feel that this pursuit through alternatives is good, as long as we can help these people to discern useful treatments from those that are useless and harmful. And in this vein, I feel it is essential that we induce people to take a critical posture toward allopathic medicine—to discriminate when medical treatment (virtually synonymous with drug treatment) is useless and harmful.

I feel this is critical for the public's health. For it's obvious that political medicine and its seeming co-conspirator, the drug industry, are more concerned with the unstinted, lavish administration of financially profitable pharmaceuticals than with the judicious and appropriate interplay of drug therapy with alternative health care methods. It's obvious that the medical establishment, as hit-man for the drug industry, can't be trusted to assure the public's welfare, and so the public had best assume this responsibility itself. My feelings about this account for my emphasis in this book on appropriate as opposed to inappropriate treatments for functionally-induced myofascopathy, and consequently, my somewhat caustic judgments of allopaths and allopathy.

The treatments I mention in this book, except in rare cases, compete victoriously with drugs in treating functionally-induced myofascopathy. I think it's safe to assume, based upon documentable history, that most allopathic practitioners will show their true colors and balk at these treatments—as a matter of principle, before having rationally evaluated them! I believe, though, that any medical practitioner who is professionally, ethically, and morally responsible will objectively assess the merit of what I have proposed.

I know drug therapy *can* be of help, especially when a patient is in intolerable pain from viciously constricted tissues or from widespread inflammation. But only for a mighty *few* patients is drug therapy called for. As for the bulk of patients, drug therapy merely masks symptoms and delays proper care. As a result, they suffer unnecessarily, and many are left with *extreme* iatrogenically-induced myofascopathy. It is for this reason that allopathic practitioners, lacking the proper orientation, education, and experience, should conscientiously bow out of the treatment and care of patients with functional spasms and functionally-induced myofascopathy. Without allopathic interference (well-intended as it may be) these patients can be brought closer to optimal health.

I hope for the sake of the public's health, that allopaths will react to my foregoing comments with a healthy self-re-evaluation. If, on the other hand, my comments are taken as an unacceptable violation of *noblesse oblige*—tough! There comes a time, dear allopath, when we all are forced to swallow a dose of our own medicine.

DENTISTS

Dentists may find the concept of functionally-induced myofascopathy useful in understanding 1) the myofascial genesis of some patients' temperomandibular joint dysfunction, 2) the importance of early *appropriate* treatment of dentally-related myofascial dysfunction, and 3) the dangers inherent in, for example, long-term masseter and pterygoid hypermyotonia.

Dentists who are interested in the conservative treatment of myofascopathy can take post-doctoral training in a chiropractic or naprapathic college. They can also take various field seminars, many of which are directed specifically toward dentists. The success of such field courses attests to the progressiveness of many dental practitioners.

Indeed, in recent years, many dentists have shown an admirable progressiveness: They have turned their attention to nutrition, and manual and electrical stimulation as alternatives to pharmaceuticals when dealing with problems such as T.M.J. dysfunction.

Chiropractors and naturapaths have used and advocated these therapies for scores of years, and for just as long, they have been persecuted for doing so. It is satisfying to see practitioners of other healing arts finally using such methods and confirming the utility of the methods for themselves. In time, I am sure these therapies will become the predominantly used methods among all types of health care practitioners. Dentists are to be praised for lending a hand in bending health care methods in this most sensible direction.

PODIATRISTS

A decline in the height of the longitudinal arches of the feet (especially if only one foot is affected) can lead to a structural imbalance. This imbalance begins at the involved feet or foot and ascends the patient's body, manifesting as articular dysrelation as far up as his atlanto-occipital junction. A fallen arch (or pronation), for example, may be accompanied by eversion of the foot and relative genu valgum of the ipsilateral knee. The involved femur will exhibit a relative decrease in height, and the sacral base on the same side will laterally flex in that direction. The patient's spine will then have an unlevel base. This will give rise to a functional scoliosis with hypertonicity of the paraspinal musculature at various points along the course of the spine. It is these points of hypermyotonia that may become the locus of myofascopathic degeneration.

21

Podiatrists can be of enormous help in correcting chronic spasms and in preventing functionally-induced myofascopathy that develops through this particular mechanism. Their therapeutic role is in correcting the patient's unbalanced pedal foundation. This may be accomplished through procedures such as proper exercise, orthopedic supports, and corrective surgery. The podiatrist's ministrations may seem remote from the problematic myofascial tissues, but their benefits to the patient can be substantial, indeed.

CHIROPRACTIC
AND NAPRAPATHIC DOCTORS

Most D.C.s and D.N.s are familiar with the problem of myofascial constrictions and the various conservative therapies for relaxing them. The medics finally have realized the major importance of this problem. For a relatively short time, they have been investigating myofascial disorders, and their work is excellent. Sadly, though, they have squandered tremendous amounts of time, energy and money. For they have through their efforts "discovered" much of what D.C.s and D.N.s have known and have used clinically for *scores* of years and which we could have taught them in a wink.

Expect no credit nor acknowledgment from these medical investigators for what we have known and used to relieve the suffering of millions! For in the mind of the average medic, although something has been *widely* and *certainly* known by everybody else, until he gets around to knowing it, it was in reality never known at all. Nevertheless, therapeutically nurturing the integrity of these tissues is an integral part of the principles and practice of both chiropractic and naprapathy. Naprapathy, in fact, might fairly be considered *the* "connective tissue specialty." Both D.C.s' and D.N.s' skills in rehabilitating myofascial tissues have contributed to their survival and success, even in the face of the incredibly oppressive and monopolistic medical establishment.

For my fellow practitioners who are seasoned in dealing clinically with this condition, I hope you will find this book a succinct and interesting review. For those who have not made the condition one of their major clinical concerns, I hope the book will entice you to study the subject in depth. I hope it will also motivate you to provide your services to the millions of people who need them; for *you* are equipped through your education and orientation to serve these millions better than any other type of practitioner.

For all of my chiropractic and naprapathic colleagues, I hope *Spasm* will help educate your patients about the nature of functionally-induced myofascopathy; and I hope it will clarify for them the role they can play in their own treatment and rehabilitation.

Warmest regards,
John C. Lowe, M.A., D.C.

INTRODUCTION

UNLESS YOU'RE A RARE EXCEPTION, YOUR BODY is stiff and tight too much of the time. One or more parts of your body, perhaps your back and neck, are uncomfortable, ache, or out-and-out hurt. You're not sure why you feel this way. You try to ignore it. When it persists too long, or when it gets in the way of things, you banish it by means of a couple of aspirin, a few beers, or some medicine a doctor has prescribed.

This can be a serious mistake. For if you continue to ignore that you have a problem, considering it "*normal* aches and pains," soothing your discomfort with alcohol or pain pills, you may damage yourself beyond repair.

You don't have to settle for this. Instead, you can live your life feeling relaxed and comfortable most of the time. Read this book. Consider your aches and pains as I view them, and try the remedies I describe. You'll then see that with a little work, you can relax yourself *deeply* and *durably*.

Spasm focuses on a part of your body that orthodox doctors have practically ignored, a part of your body that nevertheless is many people's greatest source of misery. This part of your body is the flesh that covers your bones and internal organs. It consists of the muscles that move your body and the fibrous tissues that hold your muscles together and bind them to your bones.

Spasm is about the chronic constrictions or spasms that afflict this flesh; the harm these spasms can do to you; and how you can—simply and practically—prevent or relieve these chronic spasms, or how you can make your muscles and connective tissues properly, healthily elastic.

Most people seem to think they aren't afflicted with these spasms. But leading authorities agree that chronic spasms hurt and disable the majority of people at one time or another. Moreover, there is good reason to believe that the quality of the average person's day-to-day life is drastically lowered by chronic spasms.

I want you to understand that you *can* prevent or free yourself from chronic spasms and their harm. I wrote *Spasm* both to tell you how, and, with illustrations, to show you how. *Actively* apply this information, and I'm sure your life will be both a healthier and happier affair.

—John C. Lowe, M.A., D.C.
Houston, Texas

1 CHRONIC SPASMS

IF YOU'RE LIKE MOST PEOPLE, WHEN YOU USE the word "spasm," you refer to an abrupt, violent contraction of a muscle in your leg or back. The contraction grabs you with a strangle hold and takes your breath away. As you vigorously kick, the spasm releases you. Then you sigh and complain about the horrible cramp you just had.

That type of spasm is *acute,* which means it comes and goes quickly. There's another type called *chronic.* These spasms don't shock you when they come. Instead, they insidiously grow in your muscles. They're like fat collecting around your waist. You don't notice it until one day you're dreadfully obese. Stealthily, these spasms infiltrate your muscles, usually those of your back. They're low-grade at first, but they tighten until they wrench your muscles into knotted masses. The vessels that transport blood through your knotted muscles become pinched and compressed.

After a while, the tissues the vessels supply begin to starve. And the nerves that course through your muscles are squeezed so hard that you hurt.

You may not even know you have these chronic spasms; yet they may literally choke the life out of your tissues. Eventually your muscles and the connective tissues that hold them together are left infiltrated with plastic-like scars. These scars also contract. They continue the tightening of your body into an aching knot.

It's usually this aching that brings a patient to me for help. He may describe it as a constant pain between his shoulder blades. He may say his neck, shoulder, hip, or low back has been "killing" him. Or perhaps one of his arms or legs is numb, tingles, or hurts.

He may have some basic problem such as emotional stress, arthritis, poor posture, locked spinal joints, or a nutritional inadequacy. Or he may have a whole hodgepodge of other "underlying" problems. But whatever these other problems may be, they're virtually always accompanied by chronic spasms, along with tight constrictions of his connective tissues (the fibrous tissues that hold his muscles, skin and bones together.) And it's usually these spasms and constrictions that are the source of his pain.

Early in my career, true to my training, I would direct my efforts to correcting the underlying disorder, and I assumed this would in turn alleviate the painfully tight muscles. Usually it did, albeit weeks or months after the patient and I had begun working on his underlying problem. In the meantime he suffered.

At a certain point, I began treating the patient's painful muscles first; then, secondarily, I would treat the underlying condition that seemed to be generating his spasms. The results were astonishing: the patient's pain subsided *abrupt-*

ly, and his underlying condition improved much faster than it would have otherwise.

There are good reasons for these results, and I'll explain those in the following pages. What's important here, though, is that you hear of the astounding benefits that often come from loosening your muscles and connective tissues. It's also important that you hear you can enjoy these benefits, such as freedom from daily aches and pains, through simple self-treatment, and that you may *stay* pain free.

After their initial treatments, many patients say to me, "I'm *amazed!* Absolutely *amazed!*" Or, "I just can't believe it: I've hurt for *years,* and now it's gone. It's wonderful!"

There's good reason that the typical patient is amazed. For months or years, he has endured his pain almost every day. He has been X-rayed, poked, gouged, injected, and cut —and all for naught, for the doctors have found nothing wrong! He has been insulted by the diagnosis, "It's all in your head." And he has spent too much of this preciously short life dragging through his days, zombified by pain-killing and tranquilizing drugs—and all the while, still hurting.

Then suddenly and dramatically, *relief!* And through such simple, practical methods. "Why," he asks, "doesn't everyone know about this? Why don't *all* doctors do this?" To answer these questions, I would have to expound upon the greed of the political wing of the medical-drug industry. It's a state of affairs that can shock the naive and disgust anyone with a humanitarian streak. I won't allocate an inordinate amount of space to this. But to thoroughly cover the subject of this book, I can't neglect landing a few jabs against the jaw of this industrial monster. Why? Because in its list of priorities, it places the health of the public secondary to financial profits. As a result, as I'll spell out in chapters 4, 6, and 8, the medical-drug industry is *largely* responsible for the long-range devastating effects of spasms.

Despite this public health problem, there are practical solutions to the problem of spasms and their pain. Hopefully, after reading *Spasm* and applying the methods I describe, you'll be able to relieve them yourself. But should you need help, there are plenty of health care practitioners available who are trained and experienced in the methods I describe in this book. I discuss these practitioners in chapter 8.

It's hard to calculate the percentage of Americans who suffer from chronic muscle spasms and connective tissue constrictions. There are several reasons for this. First, the victims of spasms waste millions of dollars each year for over-the-counter pain-pills to numb their pain. Their pain is suppressed, so they may not make it to doctors who can pinpoint the problem. Second, if a person with spasms does consult a doctor, the doctor is likely to be an M.D. This type of doctor is likely to miss the spasms as he looks for some "serious disease." And third, when the doctor finds nothing, he's likely to prescribe stronger pain-pills and sedatives. For at least a while, these may mask the victim's symptoms, weakening his motivation to find another type of doctor who might accurately diagnose and effectively treat the problem.

Based on my observations of patients and other people, I believe that the *vast* majority of people are affected with some chronic spasms. And I'm confident that most other doctors who *touch* their patients during examinations and treatments concur with me. What's more, people spend billions of dollars each year on pain-killers and muscle relaxers, and this testifies that tight, painful muscles aren't an isolated phenomenon from which a few uptight people anguish.

I'm not the first writer to note this problem. There is, in fact, a health-care profession called naprapathy (see chapter 8) whose main theoretical underpinning corresponds to the ideas I'm expressing. Many recently published books at least touch on the disorder. The subject of most all of these is some technique for relieving the pain from spasms. Most of the books are worth reading, and the techniques they present are worth using—*for pain relief.* This, however, to my way of thinking, isn't good enough.

Pain relief can be glorious. It's what patients most often go to doctors for, and it can be exalting as a doctor to relieve a patient's pain. But for the victim of chronic spasms, pain relief should be just the starting point. It's at least equally important that you learn to prevent spasms from returning.

In the following pages, then, I explain how to relieve your pain. In addition, though, I go beyond other writers' limp-wristed references to "chronic stress" and "nervous tension" as explanations for your spasms. I discuss the major factors that tie your body into knots and how you can control these factors. With an understanding of this, you can, if you seriously work at it, once-and-for-all eradicate your recurring spasms and constrictions.

2 MUSCLES AND FASCIA— FROM HEALTH TO HAVOC

MUSCLE, AS FAR AS I CAN DETERMINE, HAS NEVer been a particularly popular subject. People just don't seem to give it a lot of thought. Granted, there are exceptions to this. Body builders may read a great deal about muscle. There is also a small group of researchers and doctors who specialize in muscle physiology or disease. And there is, too, a comparatively small group of victims of severe muscle diseases such as muscular dystrophy. They and their family members may also learn a good bit about muscle. But for people other than these, muscle seems to hold little if any fascination. In fact, most of the people I talk with about muscle know practically *nothing* about it.

One man, for example, told me there was only one thing for sure he knows about muscle: "Mine get so sore I can hardly move if I mow the whole yard in one day." A woman told me, "Well, all I know about it is that those muscle men are *grotesque!*'' I questioned her at length, and that truly was all she knew about muscle, even though she was a college graduate.

Muscle and its connective tissues can fascinate you when you learn of the trouble they may be causing you. It's like having a surge of interest in heart physiology after you've had a heart attack. It's possible that tight muscles and connective tissues account for as much as 95% of your aches and pains, your insomnia, and your tendency to contact colds and the flu.

I wasn't aware of this when I studied muscle in college. I remember standing one day in the human dissection laboratory. My eyes were fixed on a cadaver's shoulder muscle. A fellow student had just cut it in half. Except for its grey color, I couldn't have distinguished it from a piece of rump roast of beef. I had no burning interest in muscle at the time. But it's a subject that's emphasized in chiropractic college, so we covered it thoroughly. Nowadays I'm enthralled by the subject, including its most miniscule and complex details. I'll explain the subject simply, though, so that you can easily understand it, even if you have no background in anatomy. And when you understand even this simplified version, you'll see the sense in keeping your body relaxed.

Muscles are covered, of course, with skin. But interspersed between the skin and muscle are layers of fat and a tough, white fibrous tissue. This tissue is called *fascia* (fash'/a). You've most likely seen fascia when you've pulled chicken or beef apart before cooking it. Glossy sheets of fascia adhere one muscle to another and attach muscles to other body parts such as bones. And because of its tensile strength, the fascia makes it hard to pull apart the meat and bones of the chicken or beef. Because fascia connects body parts, it's often called *connective tissue.* It plays an important role in chronic spasms, and I'll refer to it throughout this book.

Thick layers of this fascia surround and separate muscles from one another. Thinner, more delicate layers of fascia extend down into each muscle mass. Those layers wrap around and envelop the bundles of fibers that together make up the muscle mass. And even thinner and more delicate extensions of the fascia reach down into the bundles of fibers, wrapping around each fiber, separating it from, yet binding it to the other fibers. The fascia and muscle are so intertwined, in fact, that the whole complex is referred to concisely as *myofascia* ("myo" meaning muscle, and "fascia," again, meaning connecting, supporting tissue).

Because of this, when I refer to chronic spasms, I'm referring not only to sustained *muscle* contraction. I'm referring to both muscle *and* fascia. The two tissues can't be separated in that they function *together;* and when one becomes abnormal in some way, the other usually does, too.

Muscles are important in spasms because it's muscle that contracts to excess. Fascia is important because nerves travel through it to deliver impulses to muscles, and blood and lymph vessels course through it to deliver nutrients to and wastes from the muscles. Fascia is like a landscape over which railways transport raw materials to, and refuse from, a muscle factory.

When a muscle contracts, the fascia that wraps through, around, and over it is compressed. The fascia has some elastic fibers so it can stretch a bit. And as its form distorts, twisting and tightening, the vessels that course through the fascia are squeezed. This squeezing partially occludes the vessels, and they are then unable to drain away enough wastes. As a result, your muscles gradually become drenched in their own cellular wastes.

This happens to all of our muscles many times every day. Muscles contract and torque their fascia. This partially occludes blood and lymph vessels and compresses nerves in the fascia. It's usually a brief phenomenon which lasts only a few moments. It happens when you lean over in a chair to look for something in the bottom drawer of a desk. As you lean, your back muscles tighten like guy wires to keep you suspended at the necessary point in space; otherwise, upon leaning, you would topple over onto the floor. When you find what you're looking for, you sit up straight again. Your back muscles relax, the wrenching of your fascia is relieved, and the blood and lymph vessels open wide again.

In most people, though, some muscles stay contracted too tightly for too long. It's these muscles that cause trouble. They can sap the health from your body and the joy from your life—even though you don't know they are the source of your trouble.

Here's what happens: A muscle stays contracted too long (for reasons I'll discuss in chapter 4). The contraction increases the pressure inside the muscle. The pressure compresses three types of vessels—arteries, veins, and lymph channels—that course through the muscle and its fascia. The vessels may partially or even completely collapse. And this is the point at which the muscle is initially damaged.

Muscle cells must have a regular supply of fresh blood delivered to them. The fresh blood comes to muscles through arteries, and it contains oxygen, water, vitamins, minerals, proteins, fats, sugars and hormones. When the arteries to a muscle are compressed, enough fresh blood with all its health-supporting chemicals may not reach the muscle. The muscle's cells can then become nutritionally deficient for 2 reasons: 1) their nutritional supply is reduced, and 2) their nutritional needs are greater, since they're working forcefully to stay contracted.

Muscles must also be drained of "old" blood and tissue fluid. Veins drain the blood, and lymph channels drain the tissue fluids. The old blood and tissue fluids contain wastes from the muscle's cells. When the muscle is spastic and its inner pressure increases, the veins and lymph channels, like the arteries, are compressed. If the pressure is great enough, they may almost completely collapse. The wastes then back up and stagnate in the muscle. If this continues, the wastes poison the muscle.

The inadequate blood supply and wastes damage your muscle's interior by inflaming it. By-products of the inflammation irritate nerve endings, making the muscle painful when you press into it firmly. But unless you press into the muscle, you may not know it's damaged. I explain why in chapter 5.

If the inflammation persists long enough, the muscle's interior may degenerate. Its fibers may be replaced by fat and a hard, painless scar tissue. Although scar tissue itself is painless, it may cause pain. Scar tissue, you see, contracts. This is why skin puckers around an area that was cut but healed with a scar.

When scar tissue forms in one of your muscles, the scar can contract and pull the muscle into a knot. This knot, if tight enough, may compress and excite pain receptors. The muscle knot will then hurt. This knot may actually pinch arteries, veins, and lymph channels. With this, the nutritional deficiencies and waste accumulation will worsen. And eventually, the muscle may degenerate to the point that practically nothing is left but fat and scar tissue. Obviously, then, it's important to relieve your spasms before they cause scarring.

I've focused so far on the *local* ravage of spasms—how they devastate your muscles and fascia. But the destruction to your health may not end there. Other parts of your body may be even more devastated. In the next chapter, I consider some of the other possible health hazards of chronic spasms.

3 HEALTH HAZARDS OF CHRONIC SPASMS

WHEN ONE PART OF YOUR BODY BEGINS TO SERIously break down, other parts sooner or later break down, too. If, for instance, disease handicaps your kidneys, the pressure in your blood vessels may rise dangerously high, your legs and feet may swell with excess fluid, and your joints may stiffen, swell and hurt. If disease damages your heart, your shoulder and arm may cramp with spasm-like pains, your muscles may weaken, your blood pressure may drop too low, and you may pass out at times because too little blood reaches your brain.

Chronically spastic muscles are no different in this respect from any other part of your body. Eventually, your spastic muscles are likely to at least contribute to poor health elsewhere in your body. When your spasms are sparse and mild, the rest of your body may be unscathed. But when your spasms are widespread and intense, it's likely that some other part of your body will painfully mirror the disorder.

RESTLESS BUT DRAINED

Many of my patients, when they first consult me, have spasms in virtually all their back muscles. These patients typically say, "I don't understand it—I'm *too* alert, restless, and even jumpy. But at the same time, I'm tired . . . I feel absolutely *drained!*" These same patients, after beginning therapy, say they feel quite the reverse: relaxed yet energetic.

There are several reasons for these patients' paradoxical restlessness and lethargy. First, when a muscle is spastic, the chemical reactions in its cells accelerate. The muscle then uses more of the sugar, vitamins and minerals brought to it by its arteries. When *many large* muscles, such as those of your back, are spastic, a considerable bit of your energy may be depleted. This could possibly result in an inadequacy of energy-yielding nutrients in other parts of your body. This alone may not leave you feeling drained if your nutrition is good. But if your intake of vitamins, minerals and protein is marginal, as most people's seems to be, it may leave you sluggish.

Another reason spasms may make you feel drained is that they continually stimulate the "emergency" part of your nervous system. This part of your nervous system is also activated by strong emotions like anger and fear. This nervous stimulation triggers reactions in your body that prepare you for vigorous action. And while it's in operation, your energy use can skyrocket. When nerve signals continually bombard your spinal cord from spastic muscles, they may, through reflex connections, excite this emergency part of your nervous system. After staying in an emergency state for a while, your energy reserves may become exhausted, and that's exactly how you'll feel.

Another part of your nervous system can also be overly excited by spasms and drain your energy. When nerve impulses stream into your spinal cord from your spastic muscles, the impulses may travel on up the cord to the base of your brain. There, they can excite a meshwork of nerves called the reticular system. This is the part of your brain that keeps you awake and alert when it's stimulated.

When this part of your brain receives too few nerve signals, you fall asleep. When it receives too many signals (from spasms, for example) you stay wide awake; you're too alert, perhaps even nervous and jittery. Spasms can keep this part of your brain firing all night. They can keep you completely awake or in a light, restless sleep. This can leave you fatigued and cranky the next day. Sleeping pills may help put you to sleep. Naturally, though, they do nothing to alleviate the source of your insomnia and exhaustion. When you awake, you may feel more rested than usual, but your spasms are still there, and you quickly tire again.

In addition to this, spastic muscles are likely to be weak because at some point, their compressed arteries can't transport enough nutrients to the muscle cells. When, for example, we use a tourniquet to stop the blood flow to a contracting muscle, the muscle becomes fatigued in a minute or so.

Inadequate nutrition, over-excitation of your nervous system, weak muscles—all these can leave you restless yet drained. And if this is the *worst* you suffer from spasms, feel fortunate, for the potential harm is far greater.

INTERNAL DISEASE

Nerves run from each of your internal organs, like your heart and stomach, into your spinal cord, and up to your brain. These nerves carry messages to your brain about the state of the internal organs (for example, whether or not it's receiving enough blood). Your brain then transmits messages back to these organs, and the messages cause adjustments to occur in the organs (such as an increase or decrease in blood supply). Most people readily accept that this communication network exists between these organs and the brain. But for some reason they seem unaware of a similar nerve connection between internal organs and skeletal muscles and fascia.

Nevertheless, the connection exists. And because of this, disease in an internal organ can cause pain and spasms in muscles. An infected kidney, for instance, can refer pain to or cause spasms in your back muscles. You may *think* you have a spinal or muscle problem, but your back pain is a symptom of your diseased kidney.

This also works the other way around. Spastic muscles can transmit excess signals to internal organs and produce symptoms in them. Abnormal changes in skin and muscles of people's backs have been recorded, and months and even years later correlated with internal problems like coronary artery disease and peptic ulcer.

Diseased muscles and fascia, as in chronic spasms, may, then, lower the resistance of internal organs to disease. It thus appears that staying spasm-free may improve your chances of staying healthy—both on your body's muscular surface and deep within. But there are other problems that spasms may help produce in your body. Some of these may just be annoying; others may be lethal.

ALLERGIES, INFECTIONS AND CANCER

Stress is a causative thread that weaves through most diseases. But it's an especially prominent constituent of the causes of allergies, infections and cancer. Chronic spasms can be powerful stressors, and as such, they may take part in provoking these three conditions in you.

How can spasms do this? Possibly by sending endless streams of excess nerve signals up through your spinal cord into your brain. For this, as I'll explain, may tax and help impair your immune system, one of your body's main defenses against disease.

When your immune system is working right, it "recognizes" materials that are foreign to your body. It apprehends and destroys them. This is an important way your body rids itself of bacteria and potentially harmful chemicals.

But your immune system can go haywire. On one hand, it may mistake proteins from some of your own body's tissues as being foreign. It may attack and destroy them. We call this auto-immune disease. It may also mistake a protein from wheat, cheese, or seafood as being dangerous and attack it. We call your resulting symptoms a food allergy.

Your immune system on the other hand can fail to recognize and attack materials that are harmful to you. If it fails to identify and annihilate a bacterium, this microbe may infect your throat, heart valves, kidneys, intestines, your bones, and even the membrane that surrounds your brain and spinal cord. We then say you have pharyngitis, endocarditis, nephritis, colitis, osteomyelitis, or meningitis.

Some of your own body's cells can become abnormal and dangerous to you. Cancer cells are an example. They consume nutrients and multiply frantically. An efficient immune system will spot these cells and destroy them. But if it fails at this, the cancer cells may take free reign, invade and ravage your own tissues, and perhaps kill you. Cancer may, according to this view, result largely from a weakened immune system, and we can say the same about infections.

But what causes your immune system to go haywire? One cause is stress, which, as I said, spasms can induce and sustain. Stress may interfere with small areas in a part of your brain called the *hypothalamus*. When certain parts of the hypothalamus are destroyed in experimental animals, their immune systems are weakened. This finding is important, for the hypothalamus mediates emotions; it's a brain circuit that's hot when you're anxious or otherwise upset. Your hypothalamus is also the bridge to the part of your brain, called the *pituitary gland,* that regulates the secretion of hormones. Certain hormones from the pituitary gland probably play a role in producing antibodies, important personnel in your immune system's military force.

And some researchers believe that emotional upset, by disrupting the normal functions of your hypothalamus and in turn your pituitary gland, can impede your immune system's potency in reacting to harmful materials.

Spasms can, remember, excessively excite your nervous system. And by so doing, they may, with their endless volley of noxious nerve signals, help exhaust parts of your hypothalamus. In addition, your anxiety and worry over why you're so restless, irritable, fatigued, and why you hurt, may further help disrupt the efficiency of those areas of your hypothalamus. You may therefore have a double-barreled assault on your hypothalamus (both physical and emotional) and this may, via this complicated network, weaken your immune system and leave you poorly defended and susceptible to allergies, infections, and possibly even cancer.

Do chronic spasms *cause* restlessness, insomnia, allergies, infections, and cancer? Not directly. But spasms may *contribute* to all these afflictions. Whether spasms are a serious threat to your general health depends upon whether they interact with other decisive influences such as poor nutrition, emotional stress, and inadequate physical activity. But spasms are, to be sure, a stress that you can free yourself from. And if relieving your spasms reduces your general stress level, your body may be better able to resist other diseases. Staying spasm-free, then, may give you the edge—slight as it may be—in keeping yourself alive and healthy.

4 CAUSES

STUART CALDWELL IS TYPICAL OF A LOT OF PA-
tients I see. He's a hurried businessman who keeps himself
under tremendous pressure. Partly because of this (and I'll
soon explain why I say "partly") his muscles were so tight
when he first consulted me that they felt like rocks had grown
inside them.

He was impatient as I did my customarily thorough examination. He blatantly looked down at his wrist watch a
half dozen times; and he restlessly tapped his fingers on the
exam table he was sitting on.

When I had completed my exam, I gave him my conclusion: "I don't think your pain is caused by any underlying
condition like arthritis; you hurt because your muscles are
knotted with spasms."

He smirked and glanced at his watch again. "I could've
told you that."

"Well now you have an expert's reassurance," I said, with the playful tolerance I try to maintain with such smug characters. "As I treat you," I went on, "I'm going to explain how your muscles become so spastic. When you understand how they—"

"I really don't care," he interrupted, "*how* or *why* they got this way; I just want you to get rid of my pain."

"Very well," I said. "We'll get you out of your pain. We'll also go ahead and schedule further treatments for you every few weeks for the rest of the year."

"Huh?"

"Based on what I've learned about you and your problem," I said, "your spasms have causes you can correct—"

"And that's why I'm here—" he blurted out in his hurried fashion, "for you to correct them!"

"I'm sure I can *relieve* your spasms," I snapped back with equal speed. "But it's the *causes* of your spasms that need correcting. I can teach you what those causes are. Correcting them, though . . . Well, that's mostly *your* job. If you're in too much of a hurry to listen to what those causes are and to work to defuse them, then your muscles will soon be spastic again. Muscle-relaxing and sedative drugs aren't going to give you much satisfaction; and since you'll know that chiropractic treatment *really* helps, you'll be back to me or some other D.C. in short order complaining again about your pain. I don't want you coming back and telling me my treatment didn't work. You're apparently out for immediate relief of your symptoms. I just want to clarify at the outset the product you're paying for."

With our clear understanding, Stuart and I got along fine. True to his type, he took his immediate relief and left; and after three treatments, he thanked me for my help and assured me he didn't need it any more. And, again, true to his type, he was back in a month asking for some more immediate relief.

When treating patients like Stuart, I feel my clinic is somewhat like a drive-through hamburger joint. I'm providing the same type of speedy service as these "convenience restaurants." I happily accommodate most of these patients— but I stubbornly stay after them and insist that they take measures to *prevent* their spasms from reoccurring.

Eventually, most patients see the sense in what I'm saying. As they learn about and actively work to eliminate the causes of their problem, they enjoy truly *significant* relief. It takes some patients a while to reach this stage of willingness. I assume you already have, or else you wouldn't have read this far into this book. So without my preaching further about the importance of understanding the causes of your spasms, let's look at some of the more common means by which people come by their spastic muscles and constricted fascia.

TRAUMA

Most patients' chronic spasms are caused by multiple stresses, each interacting with the others to provoke or sustain the painful tension. Only in unusual cases are spasms caused by a *single* factor; but when they are, that factor is usually trauma.

Cindy Winslow, a 23 year old secretary, is a case in point. Cindy came to my clinic a year after she had fallen and injured herself while skiing. During her fall, she had hit the upper left side of her neck against a hard object. Her neck muscles drew up into spasms. She saw a general practitioner immediately. He told her she needed to see a neurologist as soon as she returned to Houston, and he gave her a prescription for pain-killers.

47

Spasm

The neurologist told Cindy that no bones were broken but that she had damaged the muscles, ligaments and nerves in her neck. Too bad, though; there was nothing that could be done. She would just have to wait. If her pain and limited movement of her neck worsened, he might have to perform surgery. And he added emphatically: "Definitely do *not* see a chiropractor—he may break your neck!"

So Cindy endured headaches, spasms, and a stiff neck for the next year—along with nausea and stomach aches from all the aspirin she was taking. At last, her boss urged her to see his chiropractic doctor. But because this D.C.'s office wasn't convenient for her to travel to, and she passed my office each day on her way home from work, she consulted me.

I examined her and took the appropriate x-rays. I found that a vertebra in her neck up close to the base of her skull was severely rotated to the left. Apparently the trauma from her fall or the resulting muscle spasms had wrenched the vertebra around. Had a doctor adjusted this vertebra, Cindy would have been relieved of her troubles promptly. But the general practitioner and neurologist she saw weren't trained in this form of therapy. By the time I saw her, scar tissue had formed, locking the vertebra in an abnormal position. And as the scar tissue had contracted, it had also distorted the positioning of other bones in her neck.

Nerve roots were stretched in Cindy's neck, causing muscle spasms in her neck and upper back. I corrected her vertebral misalignment and freed her from her spasms. I knew that the scar tissue, as it characteristically does, would tend to tighten again and reinstitute her problem. To prevent this I gave her exercises (like those in chapter 11) to keep the scars stretched. Unless she does the exercises, takes the nutrients I prescribed for her (as in chapters 14 and 15) and periodically receives spinal adjustments, her spasms will plague her by returning again and again.

Because the two doctors Cindy initially consulted didn't properly treat her, and because the neurologist misled her into avoiding proper care, her problem became chronic and complicated. But the original cause of her spasms and tissue constrictions was simple—trauma.

STRAIN

Strain, like trauma, is a *physical* cause of spasms. Obviously if you lift something that's too heavy for you, some of the muscles you use in lifting will become inflamed, perhaps some of the muscle fibers will rupture, and the muscles will hurt and contract.

But you don't have to lift heavy objects to strain muscles. I have, for example, had many students, accountants, and lawyers as patients who have come to me for strained, spastic muscles. This type of patient may strain his neck and upper back muscles by using them, hours-on-end, day-after-day, to support his head, neck and shoulders as he slumps and mantles over papers on a desk. I've also had dentists and dental hygenists as patients who have strained muscles in their right upper backs and shoulders. They usually have strained these muscles by leaning over their patients and holding their right arms up high as they work in the patients' mouths.

Factory workers gradually strain shoulder, arm and back muscles as they use the same arm, year-after-year, to shove boxes along a conveyor. Supermarket clerks do the same as they check out dozens of customers, lifting grocery items with their left arms and moving them down the counter to be bagged. Traveling salesmen strain muscles in their low backs and between their shoulders as they sit for hours each day in

49

car and airline seats that seem designed to keep chiropractors in business.

The point I'm making here is that using a particular group of muscles so much that it stays *excessively* toned can result in its being strained. The strain comes gradually. It occurs as the heightened pressure inside the tight muscle compresses the muscle's blood and lymph vessels, interfering with its nourishment and waste disposal.

STRUCTURAL IMBALANCE

One of the most common sources of this insidious, chronic strain is imbalances in the structure of your body. Most types of doctors aren't trained to recognize this source of strain. Instead, as though through some diabolical scheme, they've been brainwashed to impose drugs on you to chemically silence your body's wailing for relief from structural imbalances.

It's extremely important that you understand the problem of imbalanced structure. For chances are, if you're typical of civilized people, you're victimized by it. Let's suppose for purposes of illustration that you, like most human beings, sat in a school desk throughout most of your early years. You leaned to the right resting your elbow or forearm on the desk top, and you pivoted the weight of your body on your right buttock.

Chances are that early in your school years, the supporting ligaments of your spine and pelvis were taut and strong. Nevertheless, sitting in these desks is awkward and unnatural to our species. It distorts your pelvis, and because you do it persistently (five days a week for at least 12 years!) some of the ligaments that bind the bones of your pelvis expand and others constrict to accommodate the chronic, abnormal position of your pelvic bones.

Under ideal conditions, the human pelvis provides a level base for the spine to sit on, and the spine rises directly up into a vertical posture. But sitting in these desks *isn't* an ideal condition. And after you've been subjected to this strain for a while, leaning to the right, sitting on your right rump, your pelvis comes to slant down on its right side.

There are other habits that cause a hip to slant down on one side. Most people, for instance, spend most of their time standing with their body weight imposed on only one side, usually the right. And mothers with infants usually carry the tots on the same hip, day-after-day.

Because such habits cause a hip to slant down on one side, say the right, your spine also tends to tilt to the right. If something doesn't tug it back to the left, you'll lean to the right like the Tower of Pisa. But something does tug you back. Muscles on the left side of your back in the area of your ribs contract tightly and stay that way. They act as guy wires, pulling the leaning tower back toward the left. Your spine doesn't, of course, rigidly straighten back up. Rather, because it's flexible, it *curves* back to the left. You then have the beginnings of a scoliosis.

To keep your spine from continuing on toward your left and leaning your body too far in that direction, muscles higher up in your back on your right side chronically contract. As months and years go by, your spine curves back to the right. And as time goes on, muscles even higher up in your back, perhaps at the base of your neck and all the way up to your head, pull your spine back to the left again. What you're left with is a set of curves in your spine that keep you balanced over a gravity line. You're also left with certain muscle groups in your back chronically tightened or "spastic."

The process I've just described is both a benevolent gift of nature and a curse. It's a magnificent mechanical adaptation of your body to one of the perverted conditions we subject ourselves to in civilization. But at the same time, it's a distortion of what *otherwise* might be a well-organized organic machine, one that would function smoothly and competently without undue strain and friction. What you're left with is a machine that gives rise to aches and pains, functions inefficiently, squanders energy, and sabotages your resistance to a host of diseases.

Dr. Hugh Logan was a renowned chiropractic educator who heralded a practical approach to correcting such body distortions. He has enabled tens of thousands of chiropractic doctors to relieve the suffering of millions of patients. He wrote, "When man invents and manufactures a machine, he learns at the same time how to repair and adjust it. He watches, besides keeping it well oiled and well fueled, to see that its parts function properly. And if such working parts become bent or distorted he adjusts, straightens, or realigns them."

Chiropractors have adjusted, straightened, and balanced millions of patients' bodies, and the evidence that it can be done is available in the form of millions-upon-millions of before-and-after x-rays. The medical establishment, in its unquenchable economic thirst, has invested colossal energy, money and manpower into deceiving the public into believing the chiropractic profession has nothing of value to offer. As a result, most people with these body distortions suffer from them throughout their lives, as their bodies are poisoned with the endless array of drugs that pharmaceutical companies concoct and medical doctors promote. But such distortions *can* be corrected. And they should.

There flatly is no alternative to balancing your body's structure if you wish to be truly healthy—and *especially* if you wish to free yourself from spasms and connective tissue constrictions. To determine whether your structure is out of balance, and particularly to correct an imbalance, requires special examination procedures and corrective techniques. I've never met an M.D. who was competent at dealing with this problem, although there probably are some, since many M.D.s take post-doctoral training at chiropractic colleges. And many D.C.s don't make this structural balancing or engineering part of their practices. To eliminate structural imbalance as a possible cause of your body tension, I suggest you phone the chiropractors' or naprapaths' offices. Pointedly ask whether the doctors do structural balancing. Your best bet may be to locate a doctor who has studied and uses what's called "Logan Basic Technique." This approach is based on the teachings of Dr. Hugh Logan, whom I quoted above.

There's a lot you can do without a doctor's help to improve your body's balance. For example, stop slumping and slouching as you sit and stand. In good posture, few muscles actually take part in keeping your body erect. Your body's ligaments do most of the work. But with poor posture, many of your muscles may work constantly to keep you from falling to the ground. And these constantly working muscles may become spastic and eventually degenerate into perpetually contracting scars.

NUTRITIONAL INADEQUACIES

A "chemical" imbalance in your body can make you spastic as readily as can a "structural" imbalance. Most chemical imbalances are in some way related to poor nutrition. This is because most of the chemicals that make up your body are derived from what you eat and drink, and what most Americans eat and drink is *incapable* of maintaining balanced body chemistry.

If you don't ingest enough protein, or if you can't digest

or absorb it, your bones and their joints will eventually deteriorate. And joint disease is usually accompanied by muscle spasms. These spasms are mainly in the area of the diseased joints, such as your knees, but muscles in other parts of your body also tighten because joint disease can distort your overall structure.

A calcium or a magnesium deficiency (as I detail in chapter 14) can provoke and sustain spasms. You can become deficient in these minerals in many different ways. Your food may not contain enough of them. Eating too much lecithin to prevent fat deposits in your arteries can cause a calcium deficiency. Being bedridden for a number of days can cause your body to lose too much calcium. This is mainly because of physical inactivity, as during a hospital stay. We have many patients come to our clinic for spastic muscles who've been in a hospital for only a few days. Usually with these patients, the poverty-quality food forced upon them in the hospitals has failed to make up for the calcium loss.

A magnesium deficiency can be caused by consuming too much alcohol. It can also result from failing to eat enough dark green leafy vegetables, as the magnesium is a part of the chlorophyll that imparts the plants' green color.

Failing to eat enough vegetables, fruits, and whole grains can also slow the transit time of food through your digestive tract. The food will then deteriorate as it dwaddles through. This can leave poisonous chemical by-products to leak into your bloodstream from your colon. This may distort your body chemistry in such a way that excess muscular tension is easily provoked and maintained. This distorted chemistry is similar to that caused by too little physical activity. In both cases, your tissue fluids circulate too sluggishly, allowing toxic wastes to stagnate in your body. These wastes irritate nerve endings and can give rise to prolonged and excessive muscle tension.

DRUGS

Drugs, thrust at us by the medical-pharmaceutical industry, spearhead the list of causes of spasms and their long-range devastation. This includes both over-the-counter drugs and those your medic prescribes for you. I hastily add that drugs are a boon when used judiciously; but too often they're abused, and, deplorably, the abuse may be at the prescribing doctor's direction.

The basis of this drug problem is two fold: One, the drug industry's political and economic power has been used to indoctrinate the public with the erroneous belief that drug treatment is the *only* scientific approach to health care; and two, medical doctors and osteopaths, during their education, conveniently *aren't* educated in the use of equally (and quite often *more!*) effective non-drug therapies.

The net result: patients compliantly swallow pain-killing, muscle-relaxing, sedative, and anti-inflammatory medicines. These *may* conceal their symptoms. For most patients, though, the whitewashing is too thin, no matter how much of the drugs they swallow. The brash color of pain glares through, and the patients pursue alternative forms of treatment. When the drugs "work" for someone, life may be more comfortable for him . . . *for a while.* But as the person's symptoms lay suppressed, the underlying disorder seethes, leading to irreparable damage and, for some victims of the medical and drug industry, unconquerable pain.

Ironically, some of the drugs prescribed to suppress a patient's spasms may cause even worse spasms. Dr. Frederick Klenner, for example, a medic from North Carolina, has said: "When I see an elderly person who has a tremor, the first thing I do is check his medication. Many tranquilizers can cause tremors. If the medication is discontinued, the tremor clears up. And very few of these people really need tranquilizers, anyway." The tranquilizers to which Dr. Klenner refers belong to a group of chemicals called "phenothiazines." I've had patients consult me who were terrified by paralyzing spasms induced by taking these medicines.

A tranquilizer-like ingredient in anti-histamines may also cause abnormal muscle contractions. A woman's face, for example, began twitching and tremoring when she used antihistamines regularly. Her twitching ceased when she stopped the medication. And twenty hyperactive children were reported in one study to have developed tics from another such medicine.

Tics, tremors, and twitches can heighten your susceptibility to spasms. If you're on medicine of any sort, and you suspect it may be heightening your muscle tension, ask a pharmacist whether the medicine may be responsible. I recommend a pharmacist because he is by far better educated than the average medic in the effects of drugs, and you're more likely to receive accurate information from him. If your medicine may be causing your muscle tension, seek an alternative treatment for the symptoms the drug was intended to suppress.

It's difficult to avoid damage to muscles and fascia when drug "therapy" or "care" is used to control your spasms. You may think, despite your persistent discomfort, that your medic knows best, for he likely believes he's right as he misleads you into believing that his drugs ministration is "reasonable" health care. But there's a point at which you'll know you've whipped your medical-pharmaceutical foe; and that's when the methods I describe in this book make you feel medication isn't necessary, and when you find it takes a few moments to recall when you last took all your pills.

MENTAL AND EMOTIONAL STRESS

A source of spasms and tissue deterioration that's exceedingly hard to eradicate is mental and emotional stress. This source may be abated by moving away from the rat-race that saps the strength of many big city dwellers. But by-and-large, no matter where people go, they carry with them their inefficiencies in coping with conflicts. They're too often preoccupied with troubling matters. As they anxiously ponder their troubles, their nervous and glandular systems sizzle, and their muscles tighten in preparation for emergency action that seldom if ever comes.

What comes instead is spasms. "Normal muscle maintains a weak contraction," writes Asimov, "even when the body seems to be relaxing. This is called *muscle tone* and, in a sense, it means we are constantly exercising. Muscle tone serves to keep the individual muscles in greater readiness for contraction at short notice. The muscles begin with a headstart, so to speak. People under nervous tension usually have a more intense muscle tone and require a smaller stimulus to set them off. For that reason, they twitch and are 'jumpy.' Nevertheless, the principle [of 'muscle tone'] remains valuable, even if it can be overdone."

But when it's overdone, to "twitch" and be "jumpy" isn't the worst of it. As *nervous* tension leads to *muscle* tension, the blood supply to your muscles increases. This is to deliver more energy-yielding nutrients and to drain wastes as your muscles work at removing the source of your tension. But in "civilization," we're discouraged from using our bodies to eliminate psychological tension. Let's say you're unable to enjoy your meal in a restaurant because cigarette smoke from the adjacent table is hovering around your head. This incenses you, but you're not supposed to cold-cock the smoker. You're supposed to use your vocal cords as a substitute for your fists; and, so the story goes, the equally civilized smoker will cooperate in helping you enjoy a smoke-free meal.

But for various reasons, you may not have acquired the gumption to turn to a smoker in a crowded restaurant, explain what's bothering you, and ask for his cooperation. Instead, you may sit there in inner turmoil with your muscles knotted up as though they're trying to contain your emotional steam.

The tension from your emotional arousal can combine with tension from nutritional imbalances. And this combined tension can coalesce with tension from a structural imbalance. All this tension can then culminate in intense, sustained spasms. These spasms can become so tight and persistent that the muscles squeeze off much of their own blood supply. Then, of course, deterioration ensues.

If you find it beyond your abilities to cope with emotional stresses, I recommend you see a psychologist or a counselor. I wouldn't suggest you see a psychiatrist unless the psychologist or counselor recommends it. My reasons for saying this are contained in chapter 8.

You may find on the other hand that meditation or studies in Zen or Concept Therapy may be your best route to improved mental and emotional health. One thing is likely, though: As you use the methods I describe in the following chapters to loosen and relax your body, you will become calmer, and you may find that you face your daily stresses with greater composure.

Have I covered in this chapter *all* the causes of spasms and constrictions? Certainly not. I've merely overviewed the more common causes. You may, like many others, have some unique causes, or at least a unique *combination* of causes. But read on, for as you do, you're likely to acquire a vivid understanding of the interacting mosaic of causes of *your* body tension.

5 WHY YOU MAY NOT KNOW YOU'RE SPASTIC

PAIN SENSORS OR RECEPTORS DON'T LIE IN MUS-
cle fibers. The closest ones are embedded in the delicate fascial layers that envelop your muscle fibers. Because of this,
most diseases of muscle fibers are painless; that is, until the
fascia also becomes diseased. Chronically spastic muscles
may also be painless until their investing fascia is damaged
from the constant constrictions. And until that point, you
may know all isn't well, that you're uncomfortable or you
ache, but you may not know why.

When your muscles are spastic, recall, they impair their
own blood supply. They subsequently become inflamed.
This is partly because the impeded blood supply delivers too
little of your body's anti-inflammatory hormone, *cortisone*,
to your muscle cells. As a result, small spherical structures inside the muscle cells rupture. And upon rupturing, these
spheres release an enzyme that plays a key role in provoking
pain.

This enzyme in effect eats its way to the outside of the
cell, destroying the cell as it goes. When it's outside, the en-

zyme searches out a particular type of protein molecule. It attaches to the molecule and forces it to release from its clutch a chemical called *bradykinin*. The liberated bradykinin, like an angry bee freed from its hive, stings pain receptors, and volleys of impulses speed to your brain and register the perception of pain.

A person with spasms might suffer long bouts of emotional upset. He might therefore expend much of his cortisone in adapting to the stress. As a result, he might have too little left in his blood to fend off inflammation. He might then live with constant "muscle pain."

Another person with spasms may suffer little emotional upset. And because little of his cortisone is depleted in helping him adapt to stress, he's likely to have an *ample* supply of the anti-inflammatory hormone in the small amount of blood that reaches his spastic muscles. His muscles will resist inflammation; and despite his spasms, he might feel little if any pain.

But even if your blood cortisone level is too low, your muscles are less likely to become inflamed if your nutrition is superb. One reason for this is that vitamin E and the mineral selenium strengthen the membranes in muscle cells. Such membranes surround the spheres that hold the pain-mediating enzyme I mentioned above. And if these membranes are strong enough, they'll resist rupturing during the disturbed dynamics of a prolonged spasm. The pain-mediating enzyme may not escape and incite pain, and you may not know you have a chronic spasm.

But even when enough cortisone and nutrients reach your muscles, spasms themselves may cause pain. As the muscle fibers contract, they torque the fascia that wraps over, under, and through them. As this happens, the pain receptors, squeezed in the fascia, may fire pain impulses to your brain.

This painful firing, though, may be short-lived; for pain receptors adapt, just as cold and smell receptors do. Step into a cold shower and you may be shocked with the thought, "I'm going to freeze!" Within minutes, however, you'll feel that somehow you've warmed up. When you first walk into a stable, the horse manure may stink. But after subjecting yourself to the odor for a while, it'll seem to have vanished. Likewise with a prolonged spasm: its pain receptors may adapt so that you have no reason to think you're spastic.

But even after our receptors have adapted to cold, odor, or pain, we can re-excite them by stimulating them more intensely. If someone pours a bucket of ice water on you while you're still in what *was* a cold shower, your teeth may chatter from the cold. Stir up some of the horse manure with a stick, and you may wrinkle your nose and retreat, thinking you're about to choke from the stench. Likewise, press a finger deeply into a "painless" spasm, and you may ignite an explosive perception of pain. I've done this to patients countless times, to which they've usually responded: "Ouch! I didn't even know I had a spasm there. Why is that?"

I'd like to broadcast my answer to anyone in our tense society who thinks he may be spasm-free: Some spasms always hurt. Others only sometimes do. Still others *never* hurt. Yours may be of the latter type, and so you may have no *local* pain. Having *painful* muscles may not mean you're spastic; and having *painless* muscles may not mean you're not. Pain, then, *isn't* a consistent indicator, and considering that even painless spasms can harm you, it's important that you assess the status of your own muscles and fascia.

To do this, first read chapters 9 and 10 on pressure therapy. When you feel you understand how to properly use your hands, examine your muscles and their connective tissues—those of your head, neck, chest, shoulders, and all the rest of them down to the bottoms of your feet. You might also have someone else examine the parts of your body you can't easily reach, like your back muscles between your shoulder blades. If you have any doubts whatsoever after your self-exam, follow it with one by a properly oriented doctor, preferably (as I point out in chapter 8) a chiropractor or a naprapath.

6 IS IT SPASMS, OR SOMETHING SERIOUS?

MORE THAN OCCASIONALLY WHEN I TELL A PA-
tient, "Your problem is mainly muscle spasms," he says,
"Oh, good; it's just *spasms*. Nothing serious, eh?"

I immediately pounce upon my podium: "No. Nothing
serious in that we can *easily* rid you of the spasms. But if you
allow them to persist, and especially if you mask your
spasms' symptoms with drugs, then your problem is indeed
serious!" With such patients, I usually continue along the
following line.

Let's suppose you have a problem with your urinary
bladder. It becomes inflamed over-and-over again. Each
time, you take some medicine that suppresses the inflammation for a few weeks or months. But it flares up again.

Each time the lining of your bladder becomes inflamed, it
heals with some scar tissue. The scar tissue contracts, just as
it does in muscles. When your bladder has been inflamed
repeatedly, you'll have an abundance of scar tissue. This
tissue will pull your bladder walls in upon themselves. Eventually, the walls will constrict to a dangerous point.

Your bladder has a hole in its bottom through which a tube transports urine from your bladder to the outside world. This hole can become obstructed as your bladder squeezes in on itself from the contracting scar tissue. One complication from this is that your bladder won't be able to completely empty itself when you urinate. Urine will stagnate in the bottom of your bladder. You'll then have a cesspool inside your abdomen. Bacteria will breed in it, infect the inside of your bladder, incite more inflammation, and more scar tissue will form. You'll then have a dreadfully serious problem.

Let's suppose, to clarify this further, that the muscles around your rectum are spastic. This problem is more common than you might think. These muscles are called a sphincter. This rectal sphincter can be spastic for so long that its interior becomes inflamed. If it's persistently or repeatedly inflamed, it can become massively scarred. As the scar tissue contracts, your rectum can constrict tightly. It can tighten so much that when you pass a stool during a bowel movement, the stool is squeezed flat and coils on the bottom of your toilet like a ribbon.

When your rectum is tight, a hard or rough stool (from too little fiber in your diet) will scrape and abrade the interior of your rectum. This inflames it again, creating more scar tissue. Eventually, your rectum can become so tight that it's painful to pass even a soft stool.

The point is that prolonged spasms—because of their sequels, inflammation and scarring—are *serious,* no matter where they are located in your body. They're probably *most* serious, however, when they occur in one side of your back, a hip, or a shoulder.

Most of these muscles attach directly or indirectly to one or more vertebrae (the bones that form your spine) and to either ribs, shoulder or hip bones. When these muscles are spastic or when they contain contracting scar tissue, the vertebrae are likely to be pulled toward the other bones to which the muscles are attached, say the shoulder. As the vertebrae are pulled from their normal positions, your body's balance is thrown off. What may be worse is that the nerves emitting from between the distorted vertebrae may begin to dysfunction.

These nerves from various parts of your spine travel down your arms and legs and into your chest and abdomen. And they're responsible for transmitting vital impulses to all these structures. When the nerves dysfunction, symptoms may appear that range from headaches, to pain, numbness and tingling in your arms and legs, to internal problems such as constipation, menstrual pain, and heart dysfunction.

As I step down from my podium, I end my lecture to the patient who takes his spasms lightly: "All told," I say, "spasms may not be 'serious'—*if* they're eliminated shortly after they form. If they're not eliminated, they're as serious as any other degenerative disease. That includes heart disorders, arthritis, and even cancer, for some people have drowned and others committed suicide from the pain of spasms."

7 SHOULD YOU SEE A DOCTOR?

PATIENTS OCCASIONALLY COME TO ME COM-plaining of a painful muscle spasm when in fact they don't have a spasm at all. But it's indeed good that some of them decided to consult a doctor. Mary McCall, a former patient of mine, is a case in point. She thought she had a painful spasm. She had been bedridden for several months, having lost control of her legs after a stroke. Her medic had kept her on an anti-coagulant drug to thin her blood and prevent another stroke.

I had Mary detail for me the drugs she was taking. This is necessary when a patient has been under the care of a medic or an osteopath, for in a *considerable* percentage of cases, the patient's symptoms are caused by the medication. I ex-amined her and found she did have spasms all through her back muscles. This is a usual finding, remember, in patients who've been hospitalized.

But the swollen and painful muscle mass that was hurting Mary wasn't a spasm; it was blood that had hemorrhaged into a back muscle. She had lightly bumped the muscle against the padded corner of a chair. The muscle had hemorrhaged because the anti-coagulant drug had thinned her blood too much.

I used physical therapy and manipulation to gently disperse the hemorrhaged blood. As the swelling subsided, so did her pain. I explained to her that alpha tocopherol (a form of vitamin E) could probably keep her blood from clotting. I also told her that there are no dangerous side effects from the vitamin therapy—a noteworthy contrast with the drug therapy. She began reading nutritional literature and became a rather "health-oriented" person who, at our last conversation, refused to subject herself to drugs without first trying alternative methods.

One end of a muscle can rupture loose from its attachment. This will give rise to a large bulge when you contract the muscle, and you may think it's a spasm. Tom Lake, as an example, came to me because of a knot in a muscle between the base of his neck and his right shoulder. It had appeared about six months before when he had lifted a heavy box in the warehouse where he worked. He heard a snap in the muscle. It was painful for the following couple of weeks, but he relieved this with heat and over-the-counter pain pills.

The ruptured muscle is now weaker than its corresponding muscle in his left shoulder. It aches on occasion. The muscle should've been repaired surgically, but this would have to have been done immediately after the rupture. By the time Tom came to me, it was too late, although I did refer him to a surgeon for evaluation.

A blood clot in an artery or vein may cause the vessel to become congested, swollen and painful. If the clot is large enough, the muscle supplied by the vessel will receive too little blood. Because of this, too little oxygen, calcium and magnesium may reach the muscle. This can cause pain and possibly spasms. If a vessel is completely obstructed by a clot, part of the muscle may die. Clots, then, are dangerous and it's best to be under a doctor's care if you have this problem.

Tumors in muscle may feel and look like spasms. These are rare and usually aren't cancerous. But you definitely should see a doctor to rule out dangerous tumors.

Muscles can become laden with calcium and may even turn to bone. You may mistake the hardened part of the muscle as a chronic spasm. I know of no treatment that's uniformly effective with these cases. You should be under the care of a doctor so that, hopefully, a treatment program uniquely effective for you can be worked out. If the muscle is too painful and conservative measures don't help, the calcium or bone may have to be surgically removed.

Many patients who go to a doctor complaining of spasms are afflicted with exactly that—*spasms*. Seldom, though, are these a symptom of some deadly underlying disease. Usually the patient is just too inactive, too uptight emotionally, and has a rotten diet. There is the possibility, however—slim as it may be—that muscle knots are a reflection of some other health problem. If you're not sure and you're seriously concerned, a doctor's help can be a great aid—in fact, it may save your life.

BLACK WIDOWS AND TETANUS

If, for example, a black widow spider bites you, your muscles will quickly draw up into spasms. These aren't chronic spasms. They come on suddenly, 15 to 60 minutes after the spider injects her venom into you. You'll be nauseous, vomit, sweat, your head will hurt, and you'll have strange sensations in your hands and feet.

The bite may produce a sharp pain, but you may not be able to see the bite on your skin. You thus may not know you were bitten, and you may not have any idea why your muscles have suddenly knotted into spasms. These spiders usually bite people between April and October, and many of the victims are men bitten on their testicles or buttocks while using an outhouse. If you suspect a spider has bitten you, see a medical or osteopathic doctor immediately. It's important that you quickly have an injection of a special anti-serum. The doctor is also likely to inject you with a solution of calcium and magnesium. This may dramatically stop your muscle cramps, although they're likely to return.

If tetanus bacillus infects you, your muscles will knot up in spasms. The organism may be found on clothes and house dust. Occasionally it enters your body during surgery, skin testing, or when medicines are injected into you with a needle. It's not, then, only when you step on a rusty nail, as many people think, that you become infected with tetanus.

Within a couple of weeks after becoming infected, you may become restless, irritable and your body may hurt. But your most troublesome symptom is likely to be pain and stiffness in your jaws; hence the name "lockjaw." Your abdominal and back muscles may also become spastic, and you may have trouble swallowing. Your muscle contractions may become so intense that parts of your body hurt, and your mouth may lock shut.

If you so much as *suspect* that you're in the grip of this affliction, go immediately to an osteopath or a medic. He'll most likely hospitalize you and treat you with an anti-serum and a tranquilizer. You must take these if you intend to survive.

ENZYME DEFICIENCIES

Other spasm-provoking diseases don't appear so abruptly. There are at least two enzyme deficiencies in muscles that cause them to tighten too much. With these diseases, your muscles contract and relax normally when you're resting. But when you do anything strenuous, like walking briskly, your muscles tighten and won't relax. If you work your muscles continually, they'll become so tight that you can't move them voluntarily.

If you think you have one of these deficiencies, see a doctor. For reasons I give in the next chapter, you would best see a chiropractic or naprapathic doctor first. Both of these types of doctors should be able to diagnose your problem or refer you to a specialist who can.

HYPOTHYROIDISM

A sluggish thyroid gland can also leave your muscles too tight. When you have this problem, you'll lack energy and your face may be puffy. Your muscles may swell, stiffen and ache, and they may relax too slowly after contracting, giving you the impression that they're spastic. When you're treated for this condition, called *hypothyroidism,* your thyroid gland rather than your spasms will be the focus of the therapy. It's best to consult a chiropractor or some other nutritionally-trained doctor for hypothyroidism.

MINERAL DEFICIENCIES

Calcium and magnesium deficiencies, as I noted in chapter 4, can cause spasms; and until these are corrected, no other treatment is likely to relax your muscles for long. You may be getting enough of these minerals in your food. But even if you are, if your thyroid and parathyroid glands aren't

71

working right, your muscles and nerves may not get the benefit of the calcium. Also, if you've lost too many acid-producing cells from your stomach, you may not absorb the calcium from your food.

Your doctor should be able to determine whether you have any such problems. He may use hair and diet analyses and blood tests. Be *sure*, though, that your doctor is knowledgeable in the subject of nutrition. Your best bet is to consult a chiropractor, naprapath, or a naturopath. These three types of doctors are required to take dietary and nutritional courses while studying for their doctorates; and they may take post-doctoral courses in clinical nutrition to increase their knowledge and expertise.

I'm not one of those practitioners who try to scare you into running to a doctor every time you have an ache or pain— nor every time you have a spasm. I encourage you to unlock the shackles of dependence the medical establishment has tried to enslave you with. Learn as much as you can about your body, and learn to keep yourself healthy. There *are* times, however, when it's appropriate to see a health-care practitioner. If you have a question about the nature of your condition or how serious it is, don't hesitate to contact a reputable doctor—a chiropractor, naprapath, naturopath, osteopath or a medic.

But before you consult a doctor about your tight muscles, read the following chapter. The type of doctor you consult, as I explain, is vitally important. The right choice can make you spasm-free. The wrong choice can make you wish you had left well enough alone.

8 WHAT TYPE OF DOCTOR SHOULD YOU SEE?

SAY THE WORDS, "YOU NEED TO SEE A *DOCTOR,*" and the average American, like a conditioned Pavlovian dog, will think, "I'll call my M.D." That could be an unfortunate reflex, especially when the person needs to see a doctor for spasms.

When you're deciding what type of doctor to see for your painfully tight body, you should keep a few points in mind. First, your muscles and connective tissues are constricted, inflamed and possibly scarred. You therefore have special needs in a doctor. You need one whose concept of health includes a body structure (bones, muscles and connective tissues) that's balanced and strong yet pliant. You need a doctor who recognizes that in the long run, only a physically active and well nourished body is likely to be balanced, strong and pliant. You need a doctor who believes there are harmless ways to loosen your spastic, constricted tissues and practical measures you can use to prevent them from knotting up again. And, of *extreme* importance, you need a doctor whose education and experience has made him adept at diagnosing and treating your condition *by touching your body*. These needs leave you with two good choices: a doctor of chiropractic (D.C.) and a doctor of naprapathy (D.N.).

D.C.s and D.N.s both hold to a basic common sense belief: When your body's structure and function are kept within normal limits of balance, you won't be bothered by symptoms of disease. The aching and pain from spasms are such symptoms, and correcting your mechanical, chemical, and psychological imbalances can durably relieve your symptoms.

Chiropractors and naprapaths believe it's possible to enjoy optimal health through a health-inducing lifestyle. Specifically, we believe that if you avoid toxins in your food, water and air; if you exercise your heart and keep your muscles toned and elastic; and if you feed your body's cells all the nutrients they need, while avoiding excess fats and sugars, then your body will serve you well throughout your life. And most chiropractors and naprapaths feel that educating patients about all this is a *vital* part of a doctor's service.

If your body is spastically constricted, though, you may need potent therapy of a special kind. And it's the chiropractor and naprapath who are best qualified to provide this non-invasive, non-toxic care. The therapeutic methods of the D.C. and D.N. are for the most part the same. We both, for example, manipulate your body with our hands, may use nutritional therapy, and chiropractors may administer various forms of physical therapy.

Some chiropractors *only* adjust your spine. This alters the relation of your spine's vertebrae, discs, joint facings and supporting tissues. It also improves the physiology of these structures, and as a result, the nerves that emit from the adjusted parts of the spine may conduct impulses more efficiently. This is a valuable service, one I believe virtually all people living in civilization may benefit from if it's done often enough. This isn't, however, the type of chiropractor who can do you the most good.

As well as adjusting your spine, most chiropractors and naprapaths also manipulate (press, knead and stretch) the soft tissues around your spine and other parts of your body. Skillfully manipulating these tissues (the muscles, tendons, ligaments and fascia) elongates, loosens and relaxes them. This eliminates excessive tugging on the bones to which these tissues are attached. It also relieves the pressure from your blood and lymph vessels and nerves that run through, under and between your tissues.

To prepare your soft tissues for manipulation and to make the manipulation more effective, D.C.s may use various forms of physical therapy. We may use hot packs and special vibrators that relax, decongest and stimulate your muscles. When your tissues are severely constricted or scarred, we may use any of a number of forms of electrical therapy. Some examples are diathermy, galvanism, sine wave, ultrasound, and transcutaneous nerve stimulation (TNS).

Both D.C.s and D.N.s study biochemistry and clinical nutrition. In our practices, we may teach patients what a wholesome diet is, and we may induce them to adopt it. We may counsel patients in making specific dietary changes and recommend nutritional supplements when necessary. Our nutritional orientation is based on sound reasoning: For body cells and tissues to work efficiently, their chemistry must be balanced, and balanced body chemistry results from providing ourselves with enough of the high-quality nutrients we require.

In a discussion of this sort, the question inevitably arises,

"But what about my *regular* doctor?" My usual answer to this is, "If by your 'regular' doctor, you mean your M.D., chances are you should stay away from him, for as I'm about to point out, it may be his fault you're in your present spastic mess."

I hasten to say that there are some medics who are as well prepared to help you as most chiropractors and naprapaths are. Many M.D.s, in fact, attend chiropractic college to learn our methods. There are also medics who do research in and treat patients for the very syndrome that's the subject of this book. They have made a magnificent contribution to our understanding of the nature of this process and how to treat it. It's important to note, however, that while these investigators are medics, they don't subscribe to the "only-a-drug-can-work" orientation of the usual M.D.

We should begin discussing "the problem of the medic" where he begins—with his exams, test, and other attempts at diagnosis. The medic is indispensable for emergencies like cuts, burns, fractures and concussions. But when it comes to general health problems, and especially *optimizing* your health, he's all thumbs. He just hasn't been taught to deal with non-emergency disorders with practical solutions. This possibly explains why the medic too often can't seem to find the source of your problem, gives you some medicine to "try," and reassures you with, "Let's just watch it for a while."

As I pointed out in chapter 4, your tight, constricted condition probably has relatively simple, practical causes. Your chiropractor or naprapath will ferret out these causes from a history, exam, and, in the case of your chiropractor, perhaps x-rays or lab tests. Then he'll go about therapizing you in practical ways. If, for example, your spasms are largely due to an inadequate calcium or magnesium intake, he has been taught in nutrition courses to recognize this and to correct it with dietary changes or supplements.

The medic, however, has been taught to look for the rare, mysterious and exotic cause. Instead of nutritional deficiencies—which are rampant!—he may do a biopsy of your tissues or assay your blood. He's more likely, for example, to look for a rarity like a phosphofructokinase deficiency. If you have such a deficiency, it must be dealt with as best it can. But looking for it *first*—before looking for more common causes—is foolish. It's like neglecting to change the oil when your car begins smoking out its tailpipe, and instead cutting some of the metal out of the engine block and analyzing it for an alloy imbalance.

Medics, then, don't look first for easy-to-find, easy-to-correct causes like spinal and nutritional imbalances. They're more likely to use dangerous and painful procedures like myelograms and electromyograms in pursuit of whatever they imagine they're looking for. But if it's tough to find a medic whose approach to *testing* is sensible, it's tougher to find one who'll *treat* you sensibly.

If your spasms are due to a calcium deficiency, he's likely to prescribe muscle relaxers and pain pills. If your spasms are due to a pelvic imbalance, he's likely to prescribe muscle relaxers and pain pills. If your pain is due to plain poor posture, he's likely to prescribe muscle relaxants and pain pills. In fact, it seems that no matter *what's* causing your condition (even a phosphofructokinase deficiency), he's likely to prescribe the same type of drugs. Some medics, though, use a more "broad-scope" approach. In addition to muscle relaxers and pain pills, they also prescribe anti-inflammatory drugs and sedatives—no matter what the cause of your problem.

This conventional medical approach isn't only inappropriate—it's dangerous! These drugs only suppress your symptoms. And while you're on the drugs or as soon as you stop them, your tissues will continue to constrict, inflame, and degenerate. Your tissues may end up scarred so badly that you have a truly difficult life-long problem to manage. What's more, all pharmaceutical drugs—*all* of them!—poison you while they suppress your symptoms, and it's the damage caused by these poisons that you hear your medic whitewash with the term "side effects."

The medic's handing of spasms justifies a criticism by Robert Mendelsohn, M.D. "I believe," he writes, "that modern medicine's treatments for disease are seldom effective, and that they're often more dangerous than the diseases they're designed to treat." Let's face it—at this time, dogs rank head-and-shoulders above the M.D. as man's best friend. We can teach most dogs to help make life a happier affair for us, but trying to teach the same to the average M.D. is like trying to grow water lilies in the desert. The M.D.'s extreme business, impatience, inflated sense of self-importance, his know-it-allness and arrogance make it impossible to teach him what he should know—that he could help you best with your spasms by laying aside his prescription pad, rolling up his shirt sleeves, and *physically* treating you.

So if for one reason or another, you *must* ask your "regular" doctor to help you, talk with him about all this. Ask him to read this book. If he acts too hurried to listen, or if he seems more interested in protecting his ego than your health, go to whatever inconvenience necessary to find another doctor who'll *genuinely* help you. For your own sake, *don't* let his "expert" opinion detain you from seeking relief from another type of practitioner. One of the tragedies of modern medicine is that incalculable numbers of patients have lived and died in misery because their biased M.D.s convinced them not to pursue alternative care that may have brought relief.

If your medic becomes angry when you mention "chiropractor," you'll know you're *not* dealing with a rational fellow. Ask yourself, "Should I trust my health to a person like this—one who possibly can't spell the word 'chiropractor,' who undoubtedly knows *nothing* about such doctors, yet who loses emotional control when he hears their title, and responds like a programmed parrot with the misnomers 'quack' and 'cultist'?"

Most of the new patients I see with spasms have been under the care of numerous medics for the problem. Virtually all of them have seen a family physician, an orthopedic surgeon or a neurosurgeon. All of the patients have been taking drugs the doctors have prescribed. Some of the patients complain that they still hurt while on the drugs. Others say the drugs seem to obscure their pain, but make them feel "tired," "drained," "heavy," or "half dead." Many have said to me, "I'm just fed up with feeling like a zombie from the drugs."

Practically all these patients tell me their M.D.s never touched them. When I palpate many of these patient's bodies, their muscles are so spastic and scarred that they feel like wood. Their M.D.s never realized this because they never touched them. And when the patients didn't respond to drugs, had seen the general practitioner, the orthopedist, and the neurologist, and *still* complained of debilitating aches and pains, they were referred to medicine's last resort, the catch-all doctor for those who haven't improved through the medical cornucopia of multi-colored, multi-shaped capsules and tablets—the psychiatrist.

Most patients are insulted by this, for they know their pain is *real*. Some finally go, though, because their doctors have told them (from ignorance or deceit) that it's their final option. Usually when these patients switch from their former medics to the psychiatrist, they are merely switched from one type of drug to another . . . from, say, Robaxin, a muscle relaxer, to Valium, a tranquilizer. Now, instead of feeling like a zombie, they feel almost catatonic; and on top of the insult of being considered a "mental case," they may end up psychologically crippled by the drugs.

Some psychiatrists use drugs only as a last resort. As their first-line approach, they use psychotherapy, although they're less qualified to do so than psychologists and various types of counselors. These medics are to be admired, for even if they don't counsel away their patients' spasms, they do less harm than their drug-promoting colleagues. The worst abuse of this type of psychiatrist is that he delays proper care.

It's worth noting at this point that psychotherapy, when administered by a psychologist or marriage and family counselor, can be of great help. I believe this is because these therapists help patients to deal more effectively with conflicts that can generate constant and tremendous body tension. Some therapists also give direct instructions in physical relaxation. But if your muscles and connective tissues have undergone degeneration and scarring, you need more than psychotherapy.

There's another type of practitioner I should mention here. That's the physical therapist. These therapists usually work under the supervision and upon prescription from a medic. This is a disadvantage for at least three reasons: 1) Although the therapist is likely to know *more* about your condition than the medic, the therapist may not be at liberty to select the form of therapy you receive, this being determined by the M.D.; 2) these practitioners, in comparison with D.C.s and D.N.s, are inadequately prepared through their education and experience to administer manipulative therapy, especially in adjusting your spine; and 3) their training is limited to *physical* therapy. They have no training in clinical nutrition nor any of the related therapies you might receive through your chiropractic or naprapathic doctor. Of course, seeing a physical therapist without first seeing a doctor is a mistake. These therapists haven't been trained to diagnose and rule out dangerous conditions that may be producing your spasms.

There may be times when you need to see a practitioner other than a chiropractor or naprapath. But because these two doctors are best qualified to correct your problem, initially you should seek their aid. If you need to see someone else—a medic, physical therapist, or a psychotherapist—your D.C. or D.N. will help you determine whom it would be best for you to see.

9 PRESSURE THERAPY

PRESSURE THERAPY, TRIGGER POINT THERAPY, acupressure, reflexology, shiatsu, myotherapy—call it what you will, it can be incredibly effective. Find a tender, knotted spot in a muscle or some connective tissue; press into it so that it hurts; hold it for a period of time; and then release it and revel in the astonishing relief of your pain. It's *almost* that simple.

Over 6,000 years ago, people discovered there was a connection between certain body disorders and tenderness in certain areas of the body. The disorders vanished when the tender spots were rubbed with penetrating pressure. One of those disorders is spasms and their aches and pains. I agree with Bonney Prudden's claim that with this disorder, the therapy is 95 percent effective.

Different writers on the subject, however, don't agree about how the therapy should be applied when treating spasms. One says press hard, another says press softly. One says press only for a moment, another says prolong the pressure. How forcefully and how long you apply pressure actually depends upon: 1) whether the tender spot is a reflex or trigger point, which may be remote from the spasm; 2) whether the spot is a newly formed spasm; 3) whether it's an inflamed and degenerating spasm; or 4) whether the spot is muscle or fascia that has deteriorated into scar tissue.

Reflex or trigger points are indicated on the figures in Appendix I. These usually require only brief though firm pressure. Spasms on the other hand may require light, heavy, brief or protracted pressure. This depends on their stage of development. So that you'll understand this, let's briefly review the three stages tissues go through and consider how to perform the therapy appropriately for each stage.

Initially some of your muscles go into chronic spasms for some adaptive purpose. At this stage, your muscles may be pain-free most of the time. But when you subject the adaptively spastic muscles to some *sustained* stress, some of their fibers may contract hard enough to reduce their own blood supply. The lack of oxygen and nutrients and the quick accumulation of wastes make the muscles ache. The contractions may relax for a while as you move about during the day but tighten when you become tense again, say as you drive through heavy traffic. Your discomfort, then, waxes and wanes.

Pressure therapy at this stage need be applied only briefly, perhaps for 10 to 30 seconds. Brief pressure into a tight muscle will "milk" it, pushing out stagnant fluid and allowing fresh blood to profuse the area. At the same time, irritation of pain receptors may be relieved. The flood of noxious nerve impulses into your spinal cord will then subside. This will circumvent reflex connections with fibers that go back to and further tighten the spastic muscles. Consequently, your aching will be relieved, possibly for a long time.

Let's now suppose that some of your back muscles have been uncomfortably tight for a long time. You haven't considered this second stage to be any major health problem, although you've felt tight and tense most of the time. Your constricted muscles and fascia are inflamed and are beginning to degenerate. Once these processes begin, it's more difficult for your tissues to recover. You may detect a more prominent nodule at this stage, and you'll probably have to press harder into the nodule for a longer period of time. Be careful not to press too hard, though, or you may perpetuate or intensify the inflammation. At this stage, it's critical that you begin using heat, stretching, and proper nutrition. Otherwise you may be embarking on a course of *chronic* difficult-to-manage pain and disability.

If for months or years you've masked your pain with analgesics, muscle relaxers, or anti-inflammatory drugs, your muscles and fascia may have deteriorated to the point that they're massively scarred. Pressure therapy at this third stage may still be a great help.

The fibrous scar tissue may be scattered irregularly through your muscles and fascia. As it contracts, it may compress vessels and nerves. If so, it may produce some of the same symptoms as spasms do. To give yourself significant relief, you'll probably have to knead your constricted tissues deeply, intensely, and for long periods of time. Pressing into the scarred tissue should decongest and nourish the surviving muscle and fascia. The pressure may also stretch the scar tissue, relieving some of the compression of the vessels and nerves. Muscles in areas adjacent to the scarred tissue are likely to be spastic, and the pressure should also relax these.

At this stage, you have no choice—if you want to be healthy! You must stretch regularly and thoroughly, institute anti-spasmodic nutrition, use heat and pressure therapy daily, change your attitudes or lifestyle to mitigate your stress level, and get yourself to a chiropractor or a naprapath. The longer you delay on all of this, the more extensive your muscles and fascia are likely to be damaged.

Note this precaution: At all 3 stages of this disorder, pressure therapy can relieve your pain. In the first stage, pain relief may be all you need. But as this adaptive stage grows into the other stages, you need more than pain relief. Using pressure therapy to gloss over your pain and your degenerating tissues is no better than obscuring your problem with drugs.

Even during the first stage of spasms, don't use pressure therapy for pain relief and then ignore the stresses that generated the spasms. Spasms don't suddenly fly through an open window and attack you. They usually develop gradually because of various stresses. You *must* remove these; otherwise, as sure as the sun continues to rise, you'll suffer burdensome consequences.

With the necessary precautions, then, enjoy the relief pressure therapy can provide. To get the most from it, you'll need to know something about technique. That's the subject of the next chapter.

10 PRESSURE THERAPY—WHAT YOU NEED TO KNOW ABOUT TECHNIQUE

THERE'S AN ABUNDANCE OF BOOKS ON THE MARket that promote the use of pressure therapy. In almost every one of these, the author coins a name for his or her brand of therapy. These names are just new labels pasted on the same old bottle. Pressure therapy, trigger point therapy, myotherapy, and auto-acupressure are examples; they're only recent versions of Japanese shiatsu and Chinese acupuncture. (American doctors, you see, are among the greatest plagiarists the world has ever seen!) No matter which book on the subject you read, the body points you stimulate to relieve pain are practically the same, and so are the techniques for stimulating these points.

Whenever you use pressure therapy on yourself, your results are likely to be better if you're comfortable and relaxed. Preferably, you should be sitting or lying down. In an emergency, though, as when standing for a long time in a post office line and you feel your muscles painfully tightening, you can treat yourself while standing.

Some writers recommend you use sticks with rounded ends and other such devices to apply pressure therapy. But there are good reasons to use your fingers, thumbs and other parts of your hands. Namikoshi is a shiatsu expert. He explains that using your finger tips to stimulate sensitive spots not only increases the blood flow to the stimulated spots, but also to your fingers and hands. This renders them healthier. Moreover, he points out, there is an abundance of nerve connections between your fingers and your brain, and stimulating your fingers calms your mind. This, he suggests, is why Japanese merchants rub their hands together when dealing with a trying customer.

I believe he's right. In line with his thinking, I've reported extensive evidence in a couple of scientific papers that there is a strong relationship between good physical conditioning and mental and emotional health. More specifically, regarding hands and fingers, Morgan has found that the stronger a mental patient's hand grip, the shorter his stay is likely to be in a mental hospital. He concluded that strength of ones hand grip is a better predictor of mental health than are the standard psychological tests.

HOW DO YOU USE YOUR HANDS?

What's the best way to use your hands in doing pressure therapy? The answer to this depends upon whom you ask. One therapist says, "Always press downward firmly using the bulb of the thumb: never press forward with the tip because this can tire or perhaps injure your hand." (See figure 1.) Another says, "Pressing with the fleshy pads or bony tips of your thumbs may have little or no effect on the nerves you are attempting to stimulate. You *must* use the

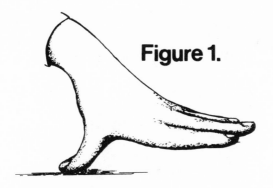

Figure 1.

nails.'' (See figure 2.) I don't think it really matters how you use your thumbs and fingers as long as you're able to apply enough pressure in the right spots.

There are some spots on your body where you won't be able to use your fingers at all. This is true of the middle of your back. Bonney Prudden recommends using a dowel to

Figure 2.

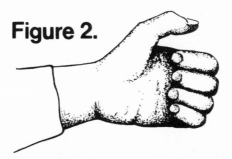

stimulate these hard-to-get-at spots. A dowel is a piece of cylindrical wood a few inches long with rounded ends. But you can just as well use your fist for most of these spots. Just reach around behind your back, and locate the sensitive spot with one of the first two knuckles on your hand. Lean against a sofa or wall with the palm of your hand, and rub the knuckle into the spot. (See figure 3).

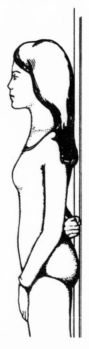

Figure 3.

HOW MUCH PRESSURE?

No matter how you use your fingers, thumbs, knuckles or even elbows, *you must press hard enough to cause pain.* Pressure therapy *isn't* superficial massage. You don't gently caress your skin. Exactly how hard do you press? Again, the answer depends upon whom you ask. One writer says, "It should be sufficient to cause a sensation midway between pleasure and pain." Another recommends that the pressure be hard enough to bring tears to a patient's eyes and to cause a bruise. This latter recommendation is extreme and unnecessary. In the past, tremendous pressure may have been necessary to break down scar tissue. But a well-trained and experienced chiropractic or naprapathic doctor uses less painful methods for loosening even the toughest scar tissues. All writers do agree, though, that the pressure you use must invoke pain, and that without the pain, there's no benefit from pressure therapy.

The pain doesn't, however, have to be excruciating. You're doing this therapy to snuff out spasms or trigger points, not life itself. When we treat patients with pressure therapy in our clinic, they may groan, moan and twist about. But the discomfort is brief, and it's well worth the relief it brings.

If you're not sure how hard to press into a sensitive spot, you might try a method Bonney Prudden has suggested. Put a bathroom scale on a table and cover it with a folded towel. Press down on the scale until it registers 15 to 20 pounds. That's about the amount of pressure needed to stimulate points on your arms and legs. You might apply 30 to 40 pounds of pressure to points in your buttocks. And on your face, you'll probably apply only about 6 pounds of pressure.

When you press into a point, if it doesn't hurt and your spasm doesn't release, try pressing harder. And if a point is unbearably painful, use less pressure. Remember, it's a trial-and-error process, and you're prospecting for what works best for *you*.

Make sure the point is sore or painful *the whole time you're pressing into it*. If while you're pressing, the pain dissipates, you may need to press harder or perhaps move your finger or thumb about to relocate the most painful part of the spot.

A few patients tell me that when they use pressure therapy, it feels like they're driving a rusty nail into their tissues. If you, like these few, are just too sensitive to the pain and feel you can't take it, there is a way to soften the pain while you're stimulating a trigger point. When you press into a spot, surround the spot with your other hand, its palm down against your skin. (See figure 4.) This can diffuse the pain so that it's tolerable. To feel how it works, find a trigger point

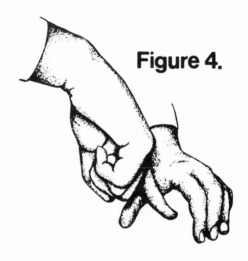

Figure 4.

and press into it hard enough to cause pain. Now, press into it again; but this time use this "diffusing" technique. Although this softens the pain, it won't reduce the effectiveness of the therapy.

Fortunately, it isn't necessary to endure the pain from the therapy for long. One writer says that you should never press into your neck for longer than three seconds. Elsewhere, such as your back, from five to seven seconds should work. Another writer says exactly seven seconds should do the job most anywhere in your body. Another recommends 30 seconds, possibly reducing the pressure once a second throughout that 30-second period of time. And yet another claims that nine minutes of pressure work best.

As I said before, trial-and-error will teach you what works best for you. In my experience, 10 to 30 seconds is usually sufficient to erase *pain*. But if you're trying to *decongest* tissues and thoroughly break up *spasms* and *constrictions,* time far in excess of 30 seconds may be necessary. With some patients who've been in particularly bad shape, I've squashed and gouged a specific constricted spot for 15 minutes a session for 10 to 12 sessions before their tissues softened. Once the constrictions let go, these patients invariably are exuberant over the relief they feel.

WHERE TO PRESS

How, though, do you know *where* to apply this pressure? Throughout most of history, instinct has guided people in using this therapy, and you're probably no exception. After all, when you're tired from walking too far, playing too much golf, slouching too long in front of the television, or sitting and typing too long, you might instinctively rub and massage the parts of your body that feel cramped or stiff.

We now have charts to guide us in using this therapy, thanks to Eastern acupuncturists and Western scientists. These charts and diagrams give us an excellent idea of which parts of our bodies to stimulate to relieve pain and spasms. The diagrams of a human body in Appendix I at the end of this book are an example. Here's how to use them. Locate on one of the diagrams the part of your body that hurts. Note the name of the muscle or muscles involved. Then find the muscle or muscles in the alphabetical list of muscles in Appendix II. The numbers that follow the name of a muscle indicate the trigger points you should stimulate to relieve your pain and possibly your spasms. You can find the location of these points on your body by noting their location on the diagrams of the bodies in Appendix 1.

Let's say, for example, you hurt in the upper part of your right hip. You turn to Appendix I and find that your pain is in a muscle called the "gluteus medius." You then turn to Appendix II and find "gluteus medius" in the list of muscles. You see that you should stimulate points 14, 15 and 16. You now turn back to Appendix I and find where these points are located in the human body. Now you merely locate these points on your own body and press into them.

Most trigger points are located in about the same place in all of us. A few points, however, may be in unusual locations, possibly as a result of injuries you've had in the past. These you'll just have to search out without the help of the diagrams and list. That's all right though, as instinct, which I pointed out, is the basis of this approach.

When you first search for trigger points in your own tissues, you may have to hunt a little. You'll know when you've found a point because it'll be exquisitely tender. When you've found a trigger point in a muscle, stimulate it for about 30 seconds, then move along the muscle at about one-inch intervals in pursuit of other points. When you find another, stimulate it, then move on looking for others. With a little experience, you'll become familiar with the location of points you usually work with, and you'll be able to go directly to them when necessary.

Most points are paired. A point on your right thigh will most likely have a corresponding point on your left thigh. Usually the *most* tender of the corresponding points will be on the same side of your body as your pain and spasms. Stimulating these more tender points usually gives the most significant relief. But if the points on the opposite side are more tender, stimulate them. This may bring the most immediate relief. It may be, of course, that your best results will come from stimulating the points on *both* sides. This is especially likely when your pain and spasms are centered or diffuse, say in the middle of your low back.

When you look at the diagrams, you'll see that a painful muscle has numerous trigger points you might stimulate. Most often, you won't want to work with all of these. Experiment and find which of the possible points brings you the quickest and most complete relief. Some of the points are easier to reach, and if easy-to-reach points bring you as much relief as the ones that are hard to get at, by all means, go for the easier ones.

If a trigger point is excruciating to press into, don't give up, concluding that you'd rather endure your spasms. When a muscle or other tissue has been tight and painful for a long time, its trigger points are likely to be extremely painful. Most likely, the *first* time you stimulate the point will be the most painful. Subsequent sessions should be less painful. In fact, if you do a thorough job with this pressure therapy, the sensitive spot may cease to be tender at all.

If your efforts don't relieve your pain and spasms, or if your relief is too short-lived, try two things: First, vary your technique. If you previously applied *steady* pressure to your sensitive spots, use a rhythmical off-on technique. Press into a spot and release it repeatedly. You might also try rubbing the spot with a circular or back-and-forth motion. The second thing you might do is stimulate a different set of trigger points, perhaps the corresponding ones on the opposite side of your body.

Your trigger points and your spasms may not overlap; that is, they may not be in the same spots in your body. You may reach around and feel a lumpy spasm in your right shoulder muscle or *deltoid*. The lump may be painless until you press deeply into it. You may, however, have felt for days or weeks a diffuse aching in the shoulder that extended all the way up into the right side of your neck. When you look at the diagrams in the appendices, you'll see that the trigger points for pain in this part of your body are located in spots remote from the lump in your shoulder. Stimulating the points should ease your pain, at least for a while; and it may release the spasm by interfering with the transmission of nerve impulses between the muscle and your nervous system. If stimulating the trigger points doesn't relax the spasm, you'll have given yourself only pain relief. In this case you should press directly into the muscle. Press until you feel pain. Persist with this direct therapy however many sessions prove necessary until the spasm is gone.

If you can't get relief no matter what you try, you may need to see a doctor who is familiar with pressure therapy. He may be able to teach you how to do the therapy more effectively. On the other hand, you may have some complicated health problem that pressure therapy simply can't conceal the symptoms of. If, for example, one of the discs in your low back is protruding, the pressure it exerts on a spinal nerve may reignite your pain as soon as you cease stimulating a trigger point. And it's critical to your well-being that you not try to obscure underlying imbalances or disease with any of the self-treatments I describe in this book. Otherwise, these treatments may do you as much harm as the painkilling drugs your medic has prescribed to camouflage your symptoms. Tools like pressure therapy serve you well *only* when you use them responsibly.

After stimulating trigger points and a muscle knot, your spasm is likely to subside. But because the muscle has been chronically tightened, it may tend to constrict again. You can, however, sustain your relief if you'll stretch the muscle after using pressure therapy. In fact, if you're to keep your body relaxed, stretching is a *necessity,* as I elaborate upon in the next chapter.

11 THE NECESSITY OF STRETCHING

"EXERCISE? UGH!" MORE THAN A FEW PATIENTS react this way verbally or with body language when I inform them they must take an *active* part in stretching their constricted tissues. "That's right," I tell them. "Like it or not, you *must* do some therapeutic exercises if you *seriously* intend to feel better. Otherwise you can resolve yourself to come to me or some other chiropractor or naprapath *frequently* for a long time . . . possibly for the rest of your life.

"But the exercises I'm talking about," I quickly add, "aren't as irksome as you may think. They require *little* time, and you don't have to work up a sweat and exhaust yourself. Remember, these are activities to lengthen and relax your tissues, not to condition you to run long-distance marathons."

"Don't need 'em, doc," executive types tell me. "I play tennis 3 times a week." Other patients assure me, "I get *plenty* of exercise at work. I'm up and down a hundred times a day, and I'm on my feet so much that they hurt!"

The movements involved in most patients' jobs can hardly be considered health-inducing exercise. They virtually never help keep patients' bodies relaxed. On the contrary, they usually induce tension.

As for tennis, racquet ball, running, and the spa or gym, they're great for conditioning your heart and toning your muscles. But they don't involve enough systematic stretching of muscles and connective tissues, and because of this, they're inadequate as anti-spasmodic exercise.

If prior to playing tennis, racquet ball or the like, you do a thorough warm-up and stretch all the major muscles of your body, this warm-up will do more to free you from spasms than the actual sport you play. Stretching is, in fact, the basis of anti-spasmodic exercises. Conversely, not stretching regularly is a sure-fire way to tighten yourself into spasms.

Unfortunately, we humans have fabricated a workaday world for ourselves in which it's inconvenient to stretch enough to keep our tissues from drawing into spasms. Our ancient ancestors awoke in the mornings and actively used their bodies. They pushed, pulled, squatted, climbed, jumped and bent all about. All parts of their bodies, from head to toe, were regularly worked to their maximum potential. Their muscles and connective tissues were contracted and stretched. This pumped fresh blood into them and waste-laden blood and tissue fluids out. This kept their tissues both toned and elastic.

Today when people awake, most of them use only a few muscles and joints to ready themselves for school or work. They use their ankles to hobble to the bathroom, a wrist and shoulder to rake a toothbrush across their teeth, and a few back and arm muscles to conceal their doughy, degenerating bodies in clothes.

Most people's muscles are hardly ever stretched their full

length. Stretching helps milk wastes from tissues, and without stretching, wastes tend to stagnate and irritate the tissue's nerve endings. This doesn't always produce distinct pain, but in most people it seems to cause at least a low-grade discomfort, the source of which is hard to identify. And people use everything from coffee and aspirin to Valium to alleviate it. While these may relieve the misery for a while, they do nothing to vanquish spasms. There simply *isn't* a substitute for regular stretching.

I envy my patients who are professional dancers. An important part of their job is to keep their body tissues stretched and flexible. To them, stretching exercises are as much a job requirement as sitting at a desk is to a secretary. But most jobs in our culture don't require us to stretch. And because of this, we must allot separate time to do stretching exercises if we're to be free from spasms.

The stretching movements of yoga are excellent anti-spasmodics. And so are those done in martial arts classes, especially tae kwon do. I encourage patients to take yoga or tae kwon do classes. But for many, it's just too inconvenient, and fortunately for our purposes, not necessary. Instead, the exercises that follow (most of which are taken from yoga and tae kwon do exercise routines) are sufficient. These stretch, elongate, and loosen the tissues of your body that in most people tend to become spastic.

Figure 5 shows the tissues that are most prone to spasms. Locate the tissues in the drawing that feel spastic to you. The numbers associated with those tissues tell you which of the exercises at the end of this chapter will lengthen and relax the tissues.

Note that the point to all these movements is to increase the distance between the two ends of a muscle group. You do this by steadily and gently moving in opposite directions the bones to which the two ends of the muscle group attach.

Using this simple principle, you can, when necessary, devise a stretching exercise to loosen any tissues that are particularly troublesome to you.

Do these exercises on a flat, padded surface with enough space to stretch your trunk and limbs in all directions. If you wear clothes, make sure these allow you to move freely. Initially you may need 20 to 30 minutes to do all the exercises correctly. Before long, though, you may need only 10 to 15 minutes. And if you're stretching only one or two muscle groups, you may stretch for only a few minutes.

Any time of the day will do, but your body will most likely be more flexible in the afternoons and evenings. If you exercise in the mornings, walk about for 15 to 30 minutes before beginning, or take a hot shower or bath. This will make you much more flexible so that you get more from the exercises.

Perform each exercise as a slow, rhythmic movement and hold the position for a moment at the end of the stretch. Don't force any movement. Gently stretch your tissues until you feel resistance. Hold the position for a moment, and then release the stretched tissues. Focus your attention on the movements you make.

Exercise twice a day for a couple of weeks. After you've loosened up—and you'll know when you have—exercise at least once each day. You'll find you're remarkably more flexible and relaxed. If you miss exercising, don't allow more than one day to elapse between sessions. When you combine these exercises with the use of heat and pressure therapy, you may be through for good with a stiff, constricted and painful body.

Figure 5.

The hatched areas indicate the tissues that are most prone to spasms. The numbers indicate which of the exercises that follow will counteract these spasms.

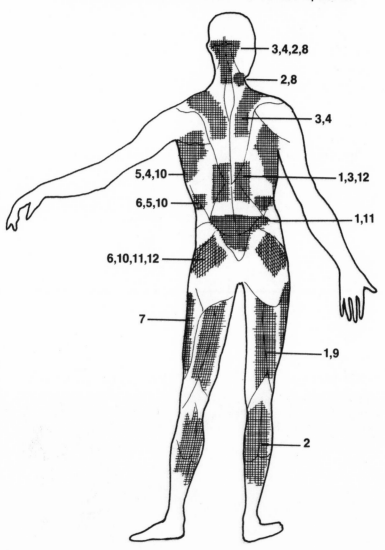

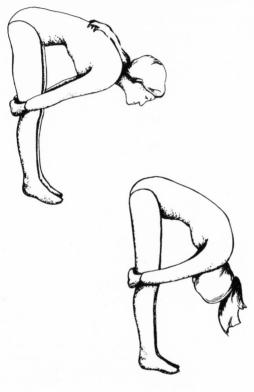

Figure 1.

Lean forward with your hands clasped behind
your thighs, knees or calves. Pull your torso
toward your knees until you feel your back,
buttocks, and thighs stretch.

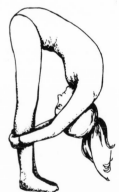

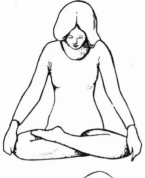

Figure 2.

Sit upright and drop your head and neck forward. Roll your head and neck to the left, to the back, to the right, and then forward again. Next, roll your head and neck in the opposite direction. In each position, drop your head and neck far enough to feel a stretching sensation on the opposite side of your body.

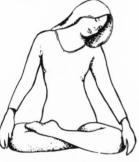

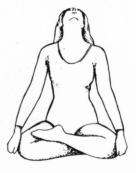

Figure 3.

Lie flat on your back. Roll your legs and hips over your head far enough so that your toes touch the floor. When you've become flexible enough, touch your knees to the floor above your shoulders.

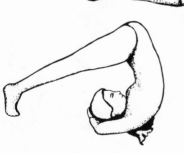

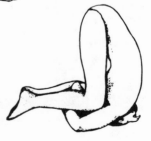

Figure 4.

Sit upright with your legs flexed in on each other. Bend forward and rotate your torso so that you touch an elbow to the opposite knee. When you've become flexible enough, bend and rotate far enough so that you touch the back of your upper arm to the opposite thigh or knee.

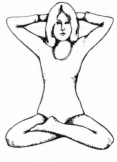

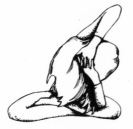

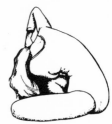

Figure 5.

Sit upright with your legs flexed in on each other. Clasp your hands behind your neck with your fingers interlaced. Pull your elbows back and lean to the right, then to the left, with the aim of touching your elbows to the floor just beyond your thigh.

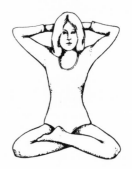

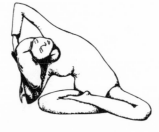

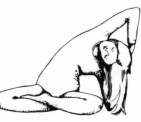

Figure 6.

Lie on your back and elevate one of your legs to 90 degrees. Lower the leg, rotating the hip, to the opposite side of your body so that you feel your low back, buttock and thigh stretch.

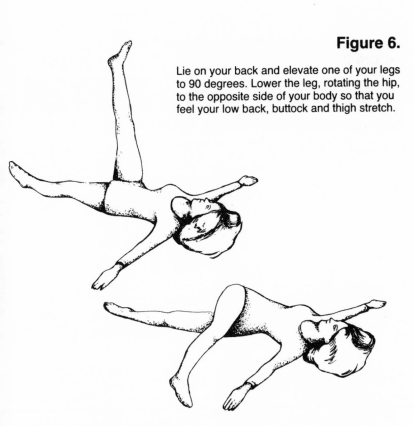

Figure 7.

Sit upright. Touch the soles of your feet together and move the outsides of your thighs toward the floor.

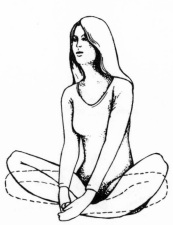

Figure 8.

Lie face down on a flat surface. Raise your head and upper torso from the surface with your elbows. First, pull your head down with your hands on the back of your head. Next, use your hands to rotate your head to the right and left.

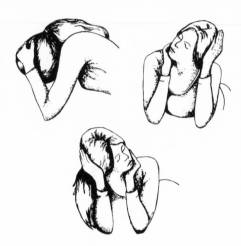

Figure 9.

Bend one leg and rest the sole of the foot against the inside of the opposite thigh. Extend the other leg and clasp your hands under the extended knee or calf. Pull your head down toward your thigh, knee or shin.

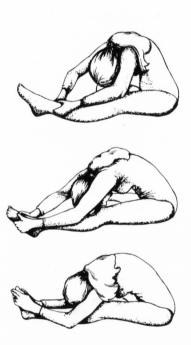

Figure 10.

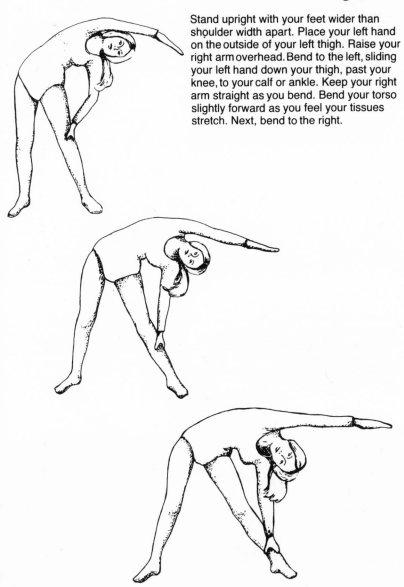

Stand upright with your feet wider than shoulder width apart. Place your left hand on the outside of your left thigh. Raise your right arm overhead. Bend to the left, sliding your left hand down your thigh, past your knee, to your calf or ankle. Keep your right arm straight as you bend. Bend your torso slightly forward as you feel your tissues stretch. Next, bend to the right.

Figure 11.

Lean forward with your hands on your hips. Move your torso in a circular motion. Lean far enough in each direction so that you can feel a stretch on the opposite side of your body.

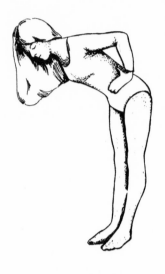

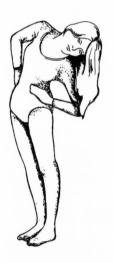

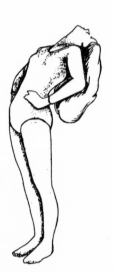

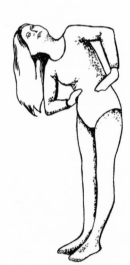

Figure 12.

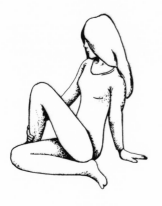

Sit upright. Fold your right leg close under your left hip. Place the sole of your left foot flat on the floor on the right side of your right thigh. Clasp the front of your right knee with your right hand. Place your left hand on the floor behind you or clasp your right side with it. Then rotate your torso to the left until you feel a stretching sensation. Repeat the exercise, turning to the right.

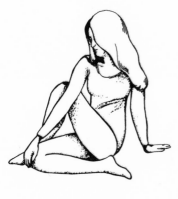

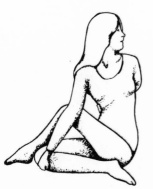

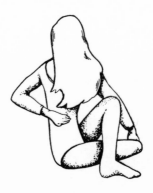

12 HOW TO USE HEAT AND COLD

AFTER I TREAT A PATIENT THE FIRST TIME FOR spasms, I pointedly instruct him: "Now and after each treatment, go home and submerge yourself up to your neck in a bathtub of hot water; and stay there until the heat sedates you."

Before powerful sedative drugs were developed, hot water was used in psychiatric hospitals to calm agitated patients. If you've ever soaked in a steaming hot tub or Jacuzzi for 10 to 15 minutes, you know well the intended effect of the hot water. The heat can be so deeply relaxing that your legs wobble when you emerge from the water. If you've never experienced this, you should. Try it when you're tired and irritable, maybe after a tense day at work or after struggling through heavy city traffic. Instead of drinking a beer or cocktail, lie in some hot water. You'll see how relaxing and, at the same time, how energizing it can be.

Heat can also relieve pain. When your back hurts or when you have sciatic pain, sit in a bath tub of hot water. Chances are your pain will vanish within 10 minutes or so, and your relief may last hours after you're out of the water.

Heat, then, can relax your muscles, calm your emotions, and relieve your pain—all anti-spasmodic effects. It's most sensible, of course, to use heat preventively. And this merely means indulging yourself, as many Japanese do, with a leisurely hot bath every day. It would best be a daily *routine,* rather than a form of "crisis therapy" resorted to after spasms have formed.

But when crisis therapy is called for, heat can be of immense help. We almost always apply moist hot packs before applying pressure therapy to a patient's spasms. The heat brings a rich blood supply into the spastic muscle and allays some of its soreness. Upon removing the hot packs, while the patient's skin is still red, we use pressure therapy and adjust his spine. This "prepping" of a patient with heat can make the difference in whether or not a defiant spasm succumbs to the other therapy. It may likewise make the difference in whether you fail or succeed with your self-treatment.

When I instruct patients to use heat at home, I always specify *moist* heat. Then comes the question, "Will my electric heating pad work?"

"Only," I answer, "if it's properly insulated so that you can moisten it." I prefer that patients use a hot water bottle separated from the skin by a moist wash cloth. Heat sedates, and many patients have fallen asleep on heating pads and have been awakened later by the pain from severe burns. The heat from an electric pad is generated continually until the pad is turned off. On the other hand, the heat from a water bottle dissipates as the water cools, and even falling asleep on the bottle isn't likely to result in a burn.

Apply heat over the tight muscle for about 5 minutes or

until your skin reddens. Then remove the cloth and water bottle. The heat will have rendered the muscle and its fascia much more flexible and relatively painless. This will make it easier for you to firmly press into and then stretch the muscle.

Some patients must use heat *cautiously,* and others would best forego it altogether. Most of these patients are elderly. As most people grow old, their blood comes to circulate sluggishly through their skin. As a result, heat isn't efficiently dispersed when it's applied to their skin. What's more, their skin becomes less sensitive. Because of this, they may not be aware that a heating pad or hot water bottle is raising the temperature of their skin to a damaging level. If you're elderly and you feel heat may benefit you, use it with a watchful eye.

Some young people's circulation is also sluggish. Usually their circulation is impaired by some type of blood vessel disease. These people, too, should be cautious, lest they burn themselves.

Others who should be careful in using heat are those with unusually low blood pressure. Blood pressure can be lowered further by heat, especially when you immerse most of your body in hot water. If your blood pressure drops too low, you'll become dizzy or even pass out. Most patients with this problem have learned about it through past experience. If you suspect that your blood pressure may be low, ask your doctor to check it for you. If it is low, talk with him about any special precautions you may need to take in using heat.

USING COLD

Because heat relaxes muscles, it may seem a paradox that cold can do the same; but cold can be anti-spasmodic when used correctly.

Touch your forearm to a block of ice briefly, say about 30 seconds, and your muscles will automatically tighten. They tighten to produce heat which warms your chilled tissues. Even though the cold tenses muscles, if you subject your muscles to cold long enough, say 10 minutes, the cold will act as a potent pain killer. And with your pain receptors numbed, you can firmly press into and gently stretch the muscle and its fascia, durably loosening them.

When you have an especially persistent and painful spasm, you may be able to break the cycle with the following method. First apply pressure therapy to the tissues. Then hold an ice cube in one hand, perhaps in a napkin or cloth so that your fingers don't become painfully cold.

Firmly rub a corner of the ice cube over the spasm. If pain is radiating from the spasm, rub the ice over your skin in the direction of the pain. Then abruptly take the ice away from your skin. Let's suppose, for example, that pain from a spastic muscle in your hip is extending down the back of your thigh. In using this form of cold therapy, you'll touch the ice to the spastic muscle in your hip and quickly slide it down your thigh over the route of the pain. If there is no radiating pain, you will just rub the ice over the spasm.

Regardless, after rubbing the ice over your skin for a couple of seconds, you'll lift the ice away and allow your skin to return to its normal temperature. This may take only 15 to 30 seconds. Repeat the procedure again and again until the muscle no longer hurts.

Note that the aim of this treatment isn't to numb the skin with the cold. Rather it's to alternate the temperature of your skin from cold back to its normal warmth. Presumably this alternating stimulation preempts the nerve pathways, and this prevents transmission of spasm-sustaining impulses from the underlying muscle. Doctors use coolant sprays such as Fluori-Methane and Ethyl-Chloride when administering this therapy. But I've used ice cubes in emergencies away from my clinic and I know they can work as well as the sprays. Ice is, of course, messier.

As with heat, you may need to be cautious with cold applications. Cold can cause tissue damage from frostbite in people with impaired circulation. But you can easily test your skin for its ability to tolerate cold. Simply rub your arm with ice briskly for 20 seconds. The proper reaction is for your skin to turn red. If instead your skin turns white, your reaction is questionable. You should consult a doctor and ask him to evaluate the adequacy of your circulation before using cold therapy—especially before you use prolonged cold applications to numb your skin.

13 HOW TO USE (AND *NOT* USE) PAIN-KILLING CREAMS AND PILLS

I OFTEN DISPENSE A TOPICAL ANALGESIC TO PA-tients whose muscles and connective tissues hurt. This is a pain-killing cream they rub on their skin. Many of them think the cream directly heals their damaged tissues. They're mistaken. All the cream does is distract them from their pain.

Most such creams contain chemicals that cause tiny blood vessels in your skin to dilate. This brings more blood to your skin and produces a sensation of heat. This sensation dominates your attention so that you don't clearly perceive pain signals generated in the tissues underneath your skin.

These creams may also contain some form of aspirin. Rubbing the substance on your skin allows some of the aspi-rin to enter your blood. This helps relieve pain much the way aspirin does when you take it orally. These liniments and creams, then, don't heal anything. And the same can be said of pain-killers you take by mouth, whether a doctor prescribes them or you buy them over-the-counter. All of them, one way or another, merely block your perception of pain.

I carefully point this out to patients, and I do so for a special reason: that is, while analgesics can give you welcome relief from pain, they can also intensify and perpetuate your problem. Pain protects your body. It tells you when your tissues are damaged. It also tells you how much you can use the damaged part without further damaging it or impairing its healing processes.

But pain can be too intense or last too long. It can annoy you so that you're irritable, you can't sleep, or you can't concentrate on work that must be done. This is when analgesics are a boon. And there's a wide array of them, from Ben'Gay, Musterole and Heet, to pills like aspirin and Tylenol and the pain-killers with dangerous side-effects that medics prescribe.

Analgesics are beneficial only when you use them to *ease* your pain. If you use them to completely deaden your pain, they can cause you more harm than good. Remember: pain is your body's way of telling you your tissues are damaged and to limit their use. When you eliminate that message with analgesics, you may stress the involved tissues and further the damage, maybe making moderate damage severe.

Most analgesics you apply to your skin don't excessively numb your pain. A cream applied over a spastic and inflamed muscle may soothe your pain. But if you stretch or contract the muscle, pain signals are likely to come through. This is the effect you want.

The greatest danger is in the use of prescription analgesics. I spend a considerable amount of time treating patients for severe damage to their tissues associated with the use of these pain-killers. Medics usually *specify* that you take a definite amount of a drug they prescribe. But people react individually to drugs. Norgesic, for example, is often prescribed for muscular pain. One tablet 4 times a day may merely reduce another person's pain so that it's tolerable. The same dosage may *totally* deaden your pain. The other patient will feel pain when he stretches his inflamed muscle. You'll feel none. You're likely, then, to overextend the damaged muscle and incite more severe inflammation. The more inflamed your muscles are and the longer they've been inflamed, the more muscle scarring you're likely to have; and the more scarred your muscles are, the harder it will be for you to loosen your body and keep it that way.

Obviously, the only sensible approach to using pain-killers is to experiment to find the dosage that best suits you— the dosage that only takes the edge off your pain. Enlist your doctor's help in finding that dosage. He should appreciate your interest in helping yourself. If he doesn't, and he arrogantly objects to your meddling in your own health-care affairs, fire him. You'll be better off to find a doctor who's willing to work *with* you.

If you use the methods I've described in this book, especially heat and pressure therapy, you shouldn't have to use analgesics, except perhaps a topical cream. But if for some reason you feel you *must* use an oral medication, use it correctly. Otherwise you may seriously harm yourself.

14 SPASMS AND NUTRITION

NUTRITION IS INTIMATELY RELATED TO MUSCLE, fascia, and spasms. Why? Because muscle and fascia, through-and-through, are formed of nutrients: proteins, fats, carbohydrates, vitamins and minerals. Muscle and fascial cells are bathed in water, itself a nutrient. And suspended in this water is an array of other nutrients.

Thousands of chemical interactions and transformations occur in muscle and fascia continuously and simultaneously. This is the means by which these tissues perform their jobs. All of these chemicals are ultimately derived from what we eat, drink and breathe; and all of their actions are triggered by enzymes that are made up of proteins combined with vitamins and minerals—more nutrients.

Many people have a tough time comprehending that their bodies are a vast organization of dynamically interacting and interchanging nutrients. There's good reason for this: Ortho-

123

dox medicine, our self-appointed authority on health and disease, hasn't yet bothered to take serious note of the fact; and therefore, they couldn't have yet passed the information on to the general public.

Some influential people in the medical orthodoxy are incredibly ignorant about nutrition. Take, for example, a former science and medical editor for the Arthritis and Rheumatism Foundation. Like other medical editors, his job was to screen manuscripts submitted for publication. He thereby had the power to determine which manuscripts would be published and would reach readers to shape their beliefs about health and disease.

This editor wrote a book on arthritis. In it, he wrote that he hoped the information he presented would put an end to the theory that arthritis is caused by a nutritional lack. He wrote further, "The scientific truth is that cortisone and hydrocortisone, the two antirheumatic hormones produced by the adrenal gland, are made from very simple substances and not from any vitamin or other foods." He might as well have written, "Hey, look how ignorant I am about the relation of nutrition to the human body." Any basic physiology textbook could've informed this editor that it's *impossible* for cortisone to be made in our bodies without vitamins, minerals, proteins, fats and carbohydrates. In fact, cortisone is made *solely* from nutrients—nothing more, nothing less.

It's not that such facts aren't available for those in orthodox medicine. It's just that at this point in history, they're involved in other things, particularly drugs and surgery. They'll come around, though, for truth is more persistent than closed minds.

Fortunately for the public welfare, facts about the relation of nutrition to our bodies has begun to seep into the more receptive minds of the medical orthodoxy. But for the time being, professional help with nutrition will have to come mainly from biochemists, nutritionists, naprapaths, naturopaths and chiropractors, the last of which have been the most open-minded and innovative in the field of nutrition and have spearheaded nutritional therapy throughout most of this century. It's testimony to their major role in the field of nutritional therapy that most companies that manufacture nutritional products for professional use consider their main market to be chiropractic doctors.

If, then, your doctor pooh-poohs nutrition, ask for his qualifications in the area of nutritional science. If he babbles something about the subject having been covered in various courses in medical school, he's most likely lying to you to keep you under his control. It's deplorable that even though he's gone through medical school, if you have a high school education, you probably know as much about nutrition as he does. The average medical doctor simply is *not* qualified to give advice on matters of nutrition.

Senator George McGovern is more qualified. After an extensive governmentally sponsored study, he wrote: "The simple fact is that our diets have changed radically within the last 50 years, with great and often very harmful effects on our health. These dietary changes represent as great a threat to public health as smoking."

And one area of our health where this threat is apparent is our bones, connective tissues and our muscles. These parts of our bodies are now dreadfully vulnerable to disease, and minor stresses and strains can debilitate them. Around the turn of the century, many people's bodies were in better shape. They worked harder physically and their nutrition was better. As a result, their tissues received more of the nutrients necessary to maintain strength and resiliency.

When these people had spasms and back pains, it was because they had lifted a load of wood or a bale of hay that was too heavy, or perhaps they had swung an ax too many

125

hours in one day. Not so with people today. Most of my patients with acute spasms and back pain tell me something like, "I just leaned over to pick up a pen I had dropped. My back has been killing me ever since." Worse yet, many patients complain that, "I just lay on the sofa for an hour or so watching T.V. When I got up I felt like a knife was stabbing into my back, and it's been like that ever since." People's tissues are so inadequately worked and so nutritionally deprived that even lying still is no protection from injury and pain.

Studies show that disorders of muscles, tendons, ligaments, fascia and spinal discs affect the quality of our lives more frequently than any other disease. Low back pain, involving these tissues, is the number one cause of employees missing work. And low back pain is second only to respiratory infections as the complaint most often taken to doctors. Spasms are involved in most all these disorders, often as a result of the disorders. Just as often, though, chronic spasms set the stage for some minor stress or strain provoking one of the disorders. Such predisposing spasms can in turn be induced, maintained, or complicated by inadequate nutrition, and correcting the inadequacies can correct the spasms and the other disorders. Let's look at some specific nutrients that may account for your spasms.

CALCIUM AND MAGNESIUM

In 1977, *Prevention Magazine* conducted a survey of its readers. The readers were asked what benefits they had received from taking calcium supplements. More than 3000 readers responded, and over half of these claimed that the mineral had relieved their spasms or cramps.

Patients can die from complications of spasms induced by a calcium deficiency. And strangling spasms may not break their hold in spite of constant dosing with muscle-relaxing drugs. A slight calcium deficiency isn't likely to kill you, but the deficiency may make you nervous, restless and tense. You may then seek the help of a psychiatrist. The average psychiatrist isn't likely to recognize the source of the problem and prescribe calcium. This is because he or she is likely to know as much about nutrition as your auto mechanic does. The doctor will probably prescribe a tranquilizer for the nervousness. And if it happens to be of a particular type (a phenathiazine derivative) you may end up with more severe spasms than an extreme calcium deficiency would cause.

A magnesium deficiency can also cause spasms. This is because this mineral must be in muscle fibers in the proper amount to trigger relaxation after a contraction. If enough magnesium isn't present, the muscle stays contracted. You then have a chronic spasm.

A low magnesium level may also intensify degeneration of muscle. This is a relatively new finding. It has been reported by Dr. Burton Altura, professor of physiology at the State University of New York. According to Dr. Altura, "We have found that when we lower magnesium, the less the magnesium content, the more the tiny blood vessels which control blood flow will contract. That to us is terribly exciting. Arteries can actually go into a contracture when the magnesium gets very, very low—or in other words, a spasm. And they'll maintain that spasm in very low concentrations of magnesium."

A spastic muscle's arteries are compressed and are thus unable to deliver an adequate amount of blood to the laboring muscle cells. If the muscles lining the arteries also are spastically contracted, even *less* blood can pass through to the muscle cells, and their nourishment may be further compromised. Magnesium, then, like calcium, must be provided in adequate amounts.

Some patients who have a knowledge of physiology may

be confused about a low calcium level causing muscle spasms. It's calcium in muscle cells that stimulates them to contract. Doesn't it follow that a deficiency of calcium would inhibit contractions and relax muscles? The muscles would relax were it not for another factor. Calcium inhibits the flow of impulses along nerves. When calcium is deficient, nerves discharge too rapidly or continually. This excites muscles excessively—even to the point of spasm.

It's worth noting, too, that you don't have to have a deficiency of calcium for the mineral to relieve your cramps or spasms. It appears to have an anti-spasmodic effect regardless. This is probably because an excess of calcium inhibits the ability of nerves to transmit impulses.

The amount of calcium and magnesium that's appropriate for you can best be determined by testing them on yourself. I would suggest that you use as a starting point, approximately 500 mg. of magnesium and 250 mg. of calcium every three hours. You may gradually increase the dosages until you feel their effect.

To absorb these minerals, you must have enough vitamin D in your system. Two or three thousand units per day have been shown to produce distinctly elevated blood calcium levels. You should be cautious with vitamin D, however, since it may cause side effects. One hundred and fifty thousand units for 10 to 14 days have stimulated oxidation of body fats and deposition of calcium in aorta and kidney. This dosage is far in excess of what you're likely to ingest daily. There is, however, the matter of individual sensitivity. Some people, few as they may be, are likely to react to low dosages—especially when taken over a period of weeks, since the vitamin is stored in fat and skeletal muscle when taken in excess of one's needs.

You can guard against such damage by taking anti-oxidants such as selenium, vitamins A, C and especially E while you're taking large doses of vitamin D. These anti-oxidants have been demonstrated to block the damaging effects of vitamin D. It's not clear what amounts of these nutrients are effective, but significantly increasing your intake while on vitamin D is probably a good idea.

You may need to take one other supplement with the calcium and magnesium to assure you absorb them. Some forms of these minerals, such as dicalcium phosphate and magnesium oxide, dissolve easily when they enter your stomach. Other forms will dissolve only when in contact with acid. If you're not sure about the forms of the minerals you have, take a capsule of hydrochloric acid or glutamic acid hydrochloride when you swallow the minerals.

If you take lecithin regularly, you may need to take additional calcium. Lecithin contains a large amount of phosphorus. When phosphorus and calcium come into contact, they combine to form a salt called calcium-phosphate. If they combine in your intestinal tract, the resulting calcium-phosphate won't be absorbed but will pass through with food residue and be eliminated as stool. If your body content of phosphorus rises too high from the lecithin, it'll combine with calcium in your blood, again form calcium-phosphate, and be eliminated in your urine. The large amount of phosphorus in lecithin can, then, leech the calcium from your body.

VITAMIN E

Doctors in Los Angeles gave vitamin E to 125 patients who had nighttime leg and foot cramps. One hundred and three of the patients completely recovered. The doctors reported, "More than half of the patients have suffered from leg cramps longer than five years and many of these had had cramps for 20 to 30 years or longer. Approximately one-fourth of the patients had cramps every night or several times a night, and in about 65 percent of the cases the cramps were severe.''

About half of these patients responded well to 300 units or less of vitamin E per day. The other half of them responded to 400 units or more. Their cramps were relieved in about a week, but they had to continue the treatment or the cramps returned.

In addition to leg and foot cramps, these researchers also used vitamin E to effectively treat rectal cramps, abdominal cramps, and cramps from strenuous exercise.

Another researcher tested the effectiveness of vitamin E in 47 men with a condition called ''intermittent claudication.'' This condition results from fat deposits obstructing the flow of blood through the arteries in the legs. The symptoms may seem simple and unimportant when they first appear. ''Typically,'' writes Dr. Wilfred Shute, ''the patient has been walking for a while—perhaps shopping, out for a stroll, or just back and forth on the job—and suddenly he or she must stop because of a severe cramp in the calf of one leg. Standing still for a short time usually causes the cramp to go away. Then walking can be resumed. In time, the frequency and severity of cramps increase, while the distance that can be covered before the cramps occur shortens.

The researcher testing the 47 men gave 32 of them vitamin E. He gave the other 15 men drugs to improve their circulation. After three months, he tested all the men to see how far they could walk without cramps. Fifty four percent of the men on vitamin E walked a little more than half a mile. Only 33 percent of the men on drugs did so.

After 18 months, 29 of the 32 men on vitamin E had an increase in blood flow to their calves. Most of the men on drugs had a *decrease* in blood flow.

There's no question that vitamin E works well in these

cases of muscle cramps due to an inadequate blood supply. It's been demonstrated in supervised double-blind, cross-over experiments as well as other types of studies. At the same time, it was demonstrated that blood vessel dilating drugs, blood thinning drugs and multivitamin-mineral preparations containing no vitamin E were of no significant help. The potential benefit of vitamin E with muscle spasms and cramps in general should be obvious.

The vitamin works in at least two ways. First, it's the chief anti-clotting agent in the blood. It prevents clots from obstructing vessels. If clots form, as they do when there are fat deposits in blood vessels, they can block the vessels enough to reduce the blood supply to muscles. Without enough blood, the muscles fail to get enough oxygen, calcium and magnesium. As a result, the muscles draw up into spasms and hurt. With enough vitamin E in your blood, existing clots are dissolved and others are prevented from forming.

But what if the blood supply to a muscle doesn't improve, as when spasms persist and compress the arteries leading into it? Vitamin E is still likely to help, even though the muscle is receiving too little oxygen from the impeded blood supply. This is because the vitamin reduces muscle cells' need for oxygen. The cells might thus be able to function as if they were receiving an adequate amount of oxygen.

Another way vitamin E works is by preventing muscles from degenerating and scarring over. In this regard, the vitamin works in conjunction with a mineral called selenium. Sheep and other livestock in certain geographical areas tend to be afflicted with what's called "white muscle disease." This disease probably corresponds to muscular dystrophy in humans. This is a condition in which muscles degenerate and are replaced by scar tissue. In livestock, the disease can be prevented by feeding the animals supplements of vitamin E

131

and selenium. It's been shown that the animals are deficient in these nutrients, and that the deficiency probably allows oxygen to destroy their muscle cell membranes. As the muscle cells degenerate, normal muscle tissue is replaced with scar tissue and fat.

Businessmen make money off *healthy* sheep; so they isolated the cure for white muscle disease—and that was that! On the other hand, special interest groups and businessmen make money off *sick* humans; so I doubt that selenium and vitamin E will be seriously investigated for some time as a way of preventing muscular dystrophy. And as a result, you're likely to hear your medic spout the illogical conclusion: "You might as well not waste your money on the stuff. It hasn't been proven that it cures muscular dystrophy." Nevertheless, these nutrients do protect the membranes around and inside muscle cells. If you're deficient in the nutrients, your muscle cells may be more vulnerable; they may easily degenerate during relatively minor but persistent spasms, become inflamed, and scar over.

If scar tissue has already formed, vitamin E may still help. Recall that scar tissue has two troublesome characteristics: it contracts and it can provoke pain. During healing, scars contract and can deform the muscle and fascia they are attached to. This may squeeze the blood vessels and pain receptors that run through the tissues. Dr. Wilfred Shute claims, "Vitamin E relaxes early scar tissue and prevents excessive scarring. The scars that are formed do not contract."

As little as 800 units a day may be effective, or as much as 3200 units may be necessary. However much you take, though, it's important to take it correctly. The vitamin is fat soluble and you absorb more when you take it with a meal containing fat. Taking it with a tablespoon of lecithin may further enhance absorption. Taking iron with the vitamin may neutralize it, so when buying a vitamin-mineral preparation, see to it that these two aren't combined in the tablets. Megadoses of vitamin C and appropriate amounts of the B complex vitamins increase the value of vitamin E. Thyroid extracts may also facilitate your body's use of vitamin E. You should consult your chiropractor, naprapath or naturopath about these extracts.

POTASSIUM

The muscles of those who eat a lot of refined carbohydrates may twitch and jerk involuntarily. The tremendous amounts of white flour, sugar and rice they eat break down to a simple sugar in their intestinal tracts. After entering their blood, some of the sugar is used for energy and much of it is stored in the liver and muscles as starch.

Whether sugar is burned for energy or converted to starch, potassium is expended in the process. As a result, the person's potassium level may drop too low, especially on occasions when he has for some reason lost a lot of fluids. Further, the sugar eater may drink a good bit of soft drinks, coffee or tea. All of these work as diuretics and wash potassium out of his body. Consequently, his potassium level may drop even further, perhaps to a critical level.

Then come the twitches. These are possibly caused by erratic and abnormal firing of nerves. Possibly more important, though, is the weakening of the muscles that accompanies a low potassium level. When you're weak all over, you're not likely to hold yourself in good posture. You may slump so much that you strain back muscles or supporting connective tissues. Or joint facings in your spine may jam. In any case, the involved tissues may become inflamed. Once your potassium level elevates highly enough so that your muscles can contract sufficiently, your strained and irritated muscles in the involved area may knot up and cause even more problems.

You may have felt the weakness of a potassium deficiency after a bout of diarrhea. If you sense a similar weakness and you suspect your muscles are weak because of a low potassium level, you may find relief in taking several hundred milligrams of potassium hydrochloride or gluconate. Moreover, you should get off and *stay* off refined carbohydrates, as I'll expound upon in chapter 16.

While calcium, magnesium, vitamin E, and potassium may be useful as anti-spasmodics, they're likely to work best when your nutrition *in general* is adequate; that is, when they're included in a wholistic nutritional program, as I point out in the following pages.

15 WHOLISM — THE ONLY SENSIBLE NUTRITIONAL APPROACH

TO GET *OPTIMAL* BENEFITS FROM A SINGLE ANTI-spasmodic nutrient, you *must* take in enough of all the other nutrients your body needs.

Proteins, fats, carbohydrates, vitamins and minerals constantly sizzle in us with incalculable numbers of interactions. The net result of all this is what we call the human body. Every nutrient in your body influences, no matter how remotely, every other nutrient in your body. And for a nutrient to serve you well, it must have available to it the other nutrients with which it interacts. This you must keep in mind if you're to *effectively* use nutrition to help you stay loose and relaxed.

Take, for example, vitamin C. Dr. James Greenwood administered this vitamin to some 500 patients. He found that it was effective in relieving their back pain from weak discs. Some patients responded better than others.

Why? One explanation is that some of the patients who didn't respond well to vitamin C weren't getting enough of some of the other nutrients they needed. My patients with disc disease and the associated spasms respond best to vitamin C when I have them also improve their protein intake. Vitamin C triggers a chemical reaction that transforms two protein building blocks, lysine and proline. These are transformed into collagen, the protein that gives strength to discs and other connective tissues. When they become strong enough, the connective tissues properly support the spine and pain is relieved. Without an adequate protein intake, the patient's body may not have enough lysine, nor enough building blocks to form proline. Without enough lysine and proline, vitamin C isn't able to stimulate the formation of collagen. And in this case, the patient isn't likely to be impressed with vitamin C. This wouldn't, however, be due to a shortcoming of the vitamin, but to a shortcoming of the patient's general nutrition.

The same can be said of vitamin C and the common cold. Someone whose nutritional status is pathetic will give vitamin C a try when his nose is dripping. It doesn't work wonders, so he concludes that the vitamin is useless. He doesn't consider that vitamin C works only in combination with the array of essential nutrients, like a fishing pole works only with a line, a hook, a sinker and bait.

Failing to understand this leads many health authorities to pronounce nutritional therapy of no value. In discussing arthritis, a Harvard medical professor wrote, "It has been established that vitamin A, vitamin B complex . . . vitamins C, E or K, when studied directly, did not alter the symptoms or course of the disease." The truth is that some of these nutrients plus others when administered alone *have* been shown to provide at least *some* relief.

Dr. William Kaufman, for example, used only vitamin

B3 with arthritis patients and made their stiff joints a bit more flexible. Other researchers have gotten similar results using vitamin B5 or pantothenic acid. But the improvements in such studies have been limited or short-lived. For anyone who understands nutritional biochemistry, this should be no surprise. Dr. Roger Williams, the biochemist who discovered vitamin B5, has commented that such benefits would probably have lasted longer if an abundance of vitamin B5 *and other essential nutrients* had been administered to the patients.

I feel that the same holds true for most any health problem we treat nutritionally, including spasms. Single nutrients are more likely to work well when they're taken along with an adequate supply of the full spectrum of nutrients. And by "full spectrum" I mean the nutrients man customarily consumed prior to his innovation of food processing and refining; before he began manufacturing gooey, plastic- and styrofoam-like "foods." The worst of these semi-foods is refined carbohydrates. These distilled sugar and starch molecules are a scourge that has produced more human casualties than any other dietary or nutritional factor in history. If you live in modern civilization, it's virtually impossible to escape this disease-inducing product of the food processing industry, and you would best read and heed the next chapter.

16 THE "CARBOHOLIC'S" SPASMS

PAULA PROVOST, A 20-YEAR-OLD SECRETARY, consulted me for pains in her low back. When I looked at her body in my exam room, I was amazed she didn't hurt *everywhere*. She was pudgy and had a boggy doughboy appearance. She reminded me of a rubber balloon half full of water.

X-rays showed that the bones of her spine were beginning to collapse. They were tilting and slumping in various directions. Her spine's supporting ligaments had lost too much tone, and her back muscles were in spasms—literally to hold up her dilapidating spine.

I talked to her about her diet and found she was a decided "carboholic"—that is, she was addicted to sugar and other refined carbohydrates such as white flour and white rice.

She was unenthusiastic when I gave her my conclusions. "You're falling apart at the seams," I said, "*mainly* because of your poor nutrition. You're starving, and your backache is your hunger pangs."

She didn't care to hear about what she was or wasn't eating, nor whether it was good or bad for her. She was polite but obvious. All she wanted was for me to get rid of her back pain. "That I can do," I explained, "but your pain will come again if you don't make serious dietary reforms."

She reformed not one jot, although I relieved her pain. But she hardly had time to get used to feeling good. Her back tightened up again and hurt. She returned to my office complaining about the inefficiency of my treatment. I told her that no matter how many times you straighten and brace a house sitting in mud, it'll continue to slip, squeak, crack and slump, and that the same applied to a skeleton with boggy supports like hers. I also loosened her new spasms and adjusted her spine so that she was once more free from pain.

In less than a week she was back in my office in pain. Again I explained to her the relation of her diet to her pain. She wouldn't budge. Instead, apparently tired of my preaching, she fired me as her doctor. She found another who would *silently* patch her up—over-and-over again.

What I lectured Paula about was irritating to her, just as the advice to give up drinking is irritating to an alcoholic. "Carboholism" is the name of her addiction, as biochemist Dr. Richard Passwater has called it. It works this way: Sucrose, also called "white table sugar," is made up entirely of simple, rapidly absorbed sugar molecules. When Paula eats this white poison, its sugar molecules rush from her intestinal tract into her blood. Her blood sugar level rises too fast. To drive it back down, her pancreas (a gland adjacent to her stomach) lavishly pours the hormone insulin into her blood. Insulin drives the sugar into her body cells.

When she overstimulates her pancreas this way day-after-day, year-after-year, it becomes "hyper." Then, even when a small amount of sugar enters her blood, her pancreas over-reacts. It ejects too much insulin into her blood. The excess insulin drives her blood sugar level too low. As a result, she craves sweet foods. The best way to satisfy her craving, so she feels, is to gulp down more white sugar or the other two refined carbohydrates, white flour and rice, or foods made from them. These kick her blood sugar level up again, and the cycle goes on.

To be enslaved to this pattern devastates the carboholic's health; and eventually he becomes plagued with mental, emotional, and physical ailments. One of the worst of these is muscle spasms in his low back, especially at the base of his spine. Most of the carboholic's problems like nervousness, fatigue or irritability occur when his blood sugar level falls too low. He can control these reactions within a few days or weeks by carefully selecting foods that don't cause a blood sugar drop.

Not so with spasms. His lousy diet has so weakened his spine's supporting ligaments and fascia that his muscles have tightened into chronic spasms to take up the slack and hold his joints together. We can relax the spasms *temporarily*. But when his body's sensors detect that his muscles' support has been withdrawn, his muscles will tighten again.

Carboholism weakens connective tissues in a couple of ways. To start with, the carboholic eats more refined carbohydrates each day than his body can possibly use. Some of the sugar is used for energy, and some is dissipated as heat. The rest—in many people, the *majority*—is stored as fat. The fat accumulates and is heavy. The extra weight burdens the supporting tissues of his spine, pelvis, knees and ankles. Over time the supports weaken.

In an athletic person with adequate nutrition, stressing ligaments strengthens them. Runners, for example, have taut yet flexible ligaments that give just the right amount of support to their low backs. On the other hand, the carboholic's own body weight, even if he's not obese, may damage his supporting tissues.

His tissues are damaged so easily because they're nutritionally deprived. They're deprived because he eats hardly anything but refined carbohydrates, and while this dietary mainstay of his is being refined, virtually *all* the nutrients are removed. Without the nutrients, the food's shelf life increases; it spoils slowly, and bugs won't eat it. Bugs apparently have enough sense to know which foods will sustain them and which won't. We can't say the same for the carboholic.

As a chiropractic doctor, I question each of my patients enough to get a good idea of what kinds of foods he or she eats. I also touch the body of every patient I examine and treat. Through this, I've become acquainted with the effects of refined carbohydrates on body tissues. The patient who has lived on carbohydrates for years is mushy to the touch. His tissues yield too easily to pressure, like squeezing a half-roasted marshmellow while it's still hot. When his skin and muscles are this much out of shape, so are his ligaments and fascia.

The patient who has lived on wholesome foods and taken nutritional supplements in most cases feels entirely different. His muscles and skin are taut. And his joints are held snuggly though pliably by healthy connective tissues. If you have doubts about this, you can easily test it on yourself and your relatives and friends. Just note the types of foods that are the person's staple, then feel of his or her waist, back, arms, and legs.

What if you're a carboholic, and your connective tissues are so feeble that your muscles have drawn up in spasms to hold your bones together. Is your prognosis necessarily a gloomy one? No. You still can firm up your connective tissues through proper diet and nutrition, combined with an adequate amount of exercise. This will remove the burden of skeletal support from your muscles. Then they'll relax. Note, though, that you can't rehabilitate your connective tissues overnight. New collagen fibers have to be formed to increase your connective tissues' tensile strength. This can take months because the metabolic rate of these tissues is slow. But the benefits are worth your patience and perseverance.

The dietary reforms I preached to Paula and which you'll have to make are clear: Don't eat white flour, white sugar, nor white rice, and eat as little as possible of any food that contains them. Eat plenty of wholesome carbohydrate foods: whole grains like oats, wheat berries, whole wheat, corn, and a variety of seeds, along with fresh, uncooked vegetables and fruits.

You can rehabilitate your tissues more expediently by immediately starting the following nutritional regimen:

1. *Protein.* See to it that you consume an adequate amount of high-quality protein each day. Some good sources are fish, poultry, rabbit, eggs and yogurt. Your doctor may recommend a protein supplement, either in powder or tablet form. Protein is essential for the production of high quality collagen. And it's necessary to form all of the enzymes that will trigger the appropriate chemical reactions.

2. *Multivitamin-mineral complex.* A multivitamin-mineral supplement along with several tablespoons of brewers yeast each day should provide enough of all the micronutrients (vitamins, minerals and trace elements) your body's chemical pathways require to regenerate healthy connective tissues.

3. *Vitamin C.* Vitamin C must be present in the cells called fibroblasts to stimulate the conversion of lysine and proline to other forms. Unless this conversion occurs as it should, collagen production will be off, and so will the quality of your connective tissues. Vitamin C, then, is critical to

optimizing the quality of your spine's supporting tissues. I recommend from 2,000 to 15,000 milligrams per day in divided doses. The higher your daily stress level, the higher your daily dosage should be.

4. *Manganese, zinc and vitamin B15.* Manganese and zinc have been determined to play key roles in the body's production of the cement that holds connective tissues' collagen fibers together. And vitamin B15 or pangamic acid has also been implicated to play a similar role. You may wish to include these in your regimen as separate supplements. The first two of these may be included in your multivitamin-mineral supplement.

Your doctor should be able to individualize a nutritional program for you if you have unusual requirements. Be sure, though, to check his credentials. Unless you're sure your doctor is qualified to help you, your best bet might be to consult a chiropractor, naprapath or naturopath.

Carboholism can be a tough addiction to overcome. It can be easier with the help of a doctor who has experience with nutritionally based problems. But whether you overcome the problem alone or with help, freeing yourself from the addiction may be the only way you can durably free yourself from spasms.

17 IF IMPROVEMENT DOESN'T COME

WHEN MOST PATIENTS COME TO ME WITH TIGHT, constricted tissues, they've already been through the medical merry-go-round. They've had the most complicated, dangerous, and advanced tests and exams, from radioactive tracings to CAT scans to exploratory surgery. If the patient hasn't had any warranted tests, I see to it that he gets them, either by doing them myself or referring him to diagnostic specialists. In any case, before starting treatment for "simple" spasms, I'm reasonably sure that no other disease accounts for the patient's pain.

Such was the case with Sam Petrol, a patient who hadn't noticeably improved during 2 weeks under my care. Therefore, when he asked me with a fretful expression, "Do you think it might be something else . . . something *really* serious?" I reassured him.

"Just because your pain is intense and tenacious," I said,

145

"doesn't mean you have some gruesome, death-inciting disease. I've seen some patients suffer more from spasms than others have from cancer. No, I *don't* think you have 'something else.' But I do agree that you have something *really* serious—a serious case of spasms. And the best thing you can do about it is to be *serious* about your treatment program."

"You can be sure of that, Dr. Lowe," he said. But I was sure of the exact opposite as I felt the rock hard muscles along his spine in his low back.

"You haven't been doing your stretching exercises regularly, have you?"

"Sure," he said. Then he shrugged his shoulders. "Well . . . when I *can.*"

"But not *regularly,* as I instructed?"

"Uh . . . no." He looked like he had been unjustly accused of a crime. "I'm too pressed for time. If I stop to exercise *every* day, I'll be *more* rushed, and then I'll be even more tense!"

"That's a poor excuse," I said. "You can do the exercises in as little as 10 minutes a day. It's a matter of priorities. Is getting healthier more important than watching the evening news on T.V.? Or scanning the newspaper? Or chatting on the phone with a friend?"

I doggedly stay after patients like Sam. In most cases, when they're not improving, they're not doing their therapeutic homework: They don't have time to exercise; the only food available at breakfast, lunch and dinner is spasmodic dietary flotsam; they "forget" to sit back for a few mintues during the day, release the "worry-wrinkles" in their foreheads and rest their chronically shrugged shoulders.

The bottom line is this: They simply aren't doing what they *must* if they're to free themselves from spasms. Sooner or later, if they're to be spasm-free, they'll have to take the bull of inconvenience by the horns.

Naturally, I concede to patients, you'll always have spasm-causing stresses you can't quickly nor easily change. So you can't divorce your monstrous spouse at the moment; you can't quit your nerve-racking teaching job until your contract expires in 6 months; you can't move from the city you hate until a job opens up in your field in the small town you love; or despite the child psychologist's efforts, your son spends more time in juvenile detention than he does at home.

In spite of all this, you *don't* have to spend your days in painful knots. Dr. S. G. Bradford has written that the degree of tension in a muscle is the sum of all the stresses bearing on the muscle at a given time. There are always some, and usually *plenty,* of tension-inducing stresses you can defuse. And the more of them you defuse, the more relaxed you're likely to be.

You can optimize your diet and nutrition; you can make stretching exercises an unvarying part of your daily routine; you can take hot baths more than once each day; you can request more tension-relieving treatments from your chiropractic or naprapathic doctor; and you can *actively* take his advice on how to cope with unique tension-provoking circumstances. You may not euphorically float through each day; but neither will you wince in pain when your eyes open each morning.

Is all this to say there's *never* "something else" wrong? No. In a few cases, the true cause of a patient's spasms and pain eludes detection, even by the best diagnostician. If you feel you're doing *everything* you should to relieve your spasms and you're not getting better, don't hesitate to talk to your doctor about reevaluating your condition.

In most cases, though, when a patient doesn't improve, the problem is one only he can solve.

18 CAN THERE BE LIFE WITHOUT SPASMS?

NATURE WAS BENEVOLENT IN GIFTING US WITH spasms. They help us adapt. Without them, life would be an even greater strain, although we would suffer for a shorter number of years.

Consider a few examples. Most people have one hip at least slightly lower on one side. Without spasms to pull their upper bodies back toward a gravity line, they would lean toward the side of the low hip. When sitting or standing, they would spend their time with the hand on the low side of the body leaning on a cane, or with the hand on the high side holding onto something to keep them from toppling over.

Consider also when someone falls on his rump and jams two adjoining joint surfaces in his low back. The muscles around the joint contract tightly so that the injured joint is immobilized until it heals. Without these protective spasms, the joint surfaces would grate and grind against one another every time the person moved his pelvis or low back. The joint might never heal properly. It might be left a mass of scar tissue, totally disabling the joint.

After using a *poorly* conditioned body to shovel all the snow off the entire driveway, or after using it to vigorously play the first softball game of the season, your strained and inflamed muscles go into spasms. These spasms remind you that you've transgressed some rules of healthy body management. And they also force you to rest the muscles until they've healed—unless, of course, you take some drug company's advice and conceal your pain with pills, in which case you may sustain some enduring damage in the form of tight scar tissue.

And finally, make beef, pork and refined carbohydrates the mainstay of your diet. In time, your blood will become so laden with fat that it'll flow through your arteries as slowly as refrigerated honey pours out of a jar. Your muscles will receive so little oxygen, calcium, magnesium and vitamin E that they'll go into spasms. You may have leg cramps at night or cramps in your chest and left shoulder that radiate down your left arm. If you wear the blinders the medical and drug industries have so carefully fitted you with, you'll use blood-thinning drugs to get more blood through your vessels to your spastic muscles. If you have good sense, you'll listen to the "quacks" and "health fanatics" and regard your spasms as a warning, then rehabilitate your body before you die of a coronary or a stroke.

Spasms, then, aren't our foe; they help us adapt; that is, until they become prolonged or chronic. When they do, they can erode our health and even shorten our lives.

But can we, in our present "civilized" circumstances, prevent spasms from becoming chronic? It can be tough doing so, for our modern lifestyle wasn't "designed" with relaxed bodies in mind. Tough as it may be, though, we *can* live in our modern world without our bodies choking the life out of us. In the chapters of this book, I've explained how. In closing, I'll summarize the ways:

1. Use your hands to examine yourself and assess the status of your muscles and fascia;

2. Resolve to do what you must to free yourself from chronic spasms, and follow through, accepting occasional backsliding as a signal to press on with even greater resolve;

3. Stay vigilant—Don't let clever drug commercials hoodwink you into believing relief awaits you in a bottle of over-the-counter pills, and don't let a medic's self-assured manner mislead you into believing that medical "science" has provided the answer in some pharmaceutical potion;

4. Stay away from doctors who were taught in school to cut, burn and poison you, and instead consult chiropractic and naprapathic doctors, as they were taught to bring health to your body through practical, harmless means;

5. Become adept at using pressure therapy along with hot packs, and possibly cold packs or ice;

6. Stretch your muscles and connective tissues regularly, especially those that tend to "knot up";

7. Improve your nutrition, and see to it that you ingest anti-spasmodic nutrients;

8. Make it a top priority to eliminate emotional and physical stresses that induce spasms and constrictions in your muscles and fascia.

If you invest your time and energy in all this, are you *guaranteed* to be free from chronic spasms? No! Like Burr-Rabbit, we've been thrown into a briar batch, a gnarled tangle of prickly damned-if-you-do, damned-if-you-don't conflicts. But you can *greatly* increase your chances of residing in this barbed mess without knotting up in tenacious spasms. This requires that you *convict* yourself to effectively deal with the stresses that induce chronic spasms, and, come hell-or-high-water, *stick* to your convictions. Your conviction in itself can be anti-spasmodic, as you experience what G. Gordon Liddy phrases a "deeper appreciation of the extraordinary power of the human will."

Yes, then; you're likely to be rewarded if you'll *actively* and *persistently* follow my recommendations. Your body may work right for the first time in a long time—all your muscles may go into spasms when it's adaptive for you, and then "tone down" to their relaxed state when the value of the spasms has passed. Now, rise from your derriere and get to work applying the contents of this book. It's truly worth it, considering the painfully tight alternative!

Appendix I
Trigger Points

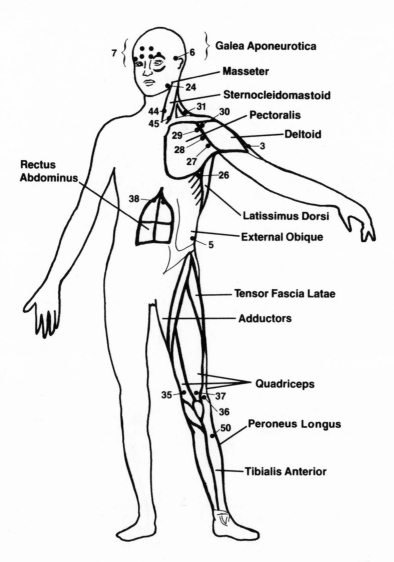

Galea Aponeurotica

7

6

Masseter

24

Sternocleidomastoid

44
45

31

30

Pectoralis

29

28

27

Deltoid

3

26

Rectus
Abdominus

38

Latissimus Dorsi

External Obique

5

Tensor Fascia Latae

Adductors

Quadriceps

35

37

36

Peroneus Longus

50

Tibialis Anterior

Appendix I
Trigger Points

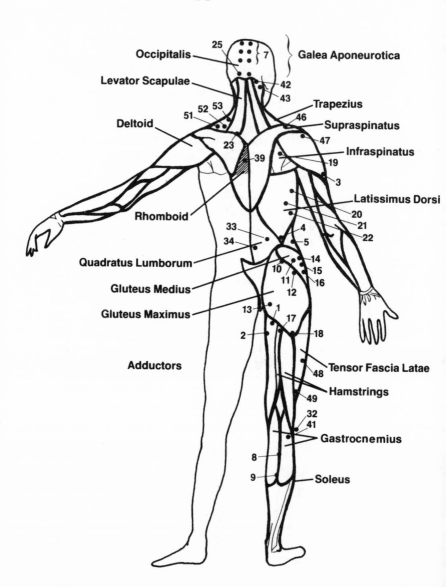

Occipitalis — 25 7 — Galea Aponeurotica

Levator Scapulae — 42 43

52 53 Trapezius
51 46
Deltoid — Supraspinatus
23 47
39 Infraspinatus
19
3

Latissimus Dorsi
20
21
22

Rhomboid

33 4
34 5
Quadratus Lumborum 14
10 15
Gluteus Medius 11 16
12
Gluteus Maximus 13 1
17
2 18

Adductors Tensor Fascia Latae
48
Hamstrings
49
32
41
Gastrocnemius
8
9 Soleus

Appendix II
Muscles and Trigger Point Numbers

Muscles	Trigger Numbers
Adductors	1,2
Deltoid	3
External oblique	4,5
Galea aponeurotica	6,7
Gastrocnemius	8,9
Gluteus maximus	10,11,12,13
Gluteus medius	14,15,16
Hamstrings	17,18
Infraspinatus	19
Latissimus dorsi	20,21,22
Levator scapulae	23
Masseter	24
Occipitalis	25
Pectoralis	26,27,28,29,30,31
Peroneus longus	32
Quadratus lumborum	33,34
Quadriceps	35,36,37
Rectus abdominus	38
Rhomboid	39
Soleus	41
Sternocleidomastoid	42,43,44,45
Supraspinatus	46,47
Tensor fascia latae	48,49
Tibialis anterior	50
Trapezius	31,51,52,53

SELECTED REFERENCES

YOU MAY WISH TO LEARN MORE ABOUT CHRONIC spasms. If so, it would be to your advantage to dip into some of the papers, articles, and books I've listed in this section. Dip, however, questioningly and skeptically, and form your ideas about this subject from *your* interpretation of the materials you read. To arrive at reasonable conclusions, I suggest that you read a fair cross-sampling of the various sources I've listed.

Health care professionals and scientists will most likely want to read primary sources; that is, journal papers in which research reports are first published. If you're not a member of one of these groups, you may or may not wish to consult scientific journals. If you wish to but don't know how, the librarians at biomedical libraries, like librarians most everywhere, will help you locate the papers you wish to read. One reason you may want to obtain some of these papers is to have your doctor read them, as this is more likely to induce him or her to see things your way and treat you as *you* see fit. You may wish, though, to expand your knowledge of chronic spasms by reading secondary sources. These consist mainly of magazine articles and books that contain writers' interpretations of primary sources.

The references I've listed certainly don't exhaust the publications that touch on or directly address the subject of this book. The list isn't an attempt to form a MEDLARS comprehensive compilation of relevant biomedical literature. Instead, it's a *sampling* of the available literature relevant to the subject of chronic spasms. This sampling is some of the main literature I've used in conjunction with my clinical experience to form my opinions on the subject.

How can you tell which of the following references are likely to interest and help you? You'll know from the titles of the papers, articles, books. Consider this for an example: An article entitled "Helping Yourself with Vitamin E" will obviously appeal to the reader with a different educational background than an article titled "Interstitial Myofibrositis."

It's perfectly alright, of course, if you read nothing more about the subject of chronic spasms than what I've written in the pages of this book. If *feeling better* is your goal, you may need to read nothing more; just actively apply the information and instructions I've given you. Some people, however, feel better only when they know a great deal about some phenomenon that affects their health. For those of you who are this way (who incidentally are cut from the same cloth as I) reading some of the references listed in this section may help you feel quite well, indeed.

Adams, R. A., "The spasm and stiffness syndromes," in *Harrison's Principles of Internal Medicine,* by G. W. Thorn, R. A. Adams, E. Braunwald, K. J. Isselbacher, R. G. Petersdorf (editors), New York, McGraw-Hill Book Co., 1977, pp. 2001-2005.

Adams, R. D., *Diseases of Muscle: A Study in Pathology.* New York, Harper and Row, Publishers, 3rd edition, 1975.

Anderson, T. W., "A double-blind trial of vitamin E in angina pectoris," *The American Journal of Clinical Nutrition,* vol. 27, Oct., 1974, pp. 1174-1178.

Awad, E. A., "Interstitial myofibrositis: hypothesis of the mechanism," *Archives of Physical Medicine,* vol. 54, 1973, pp. 440-453.

Basmajian, J. V., "Cyclobenzaprine hydrochloride effect on skeletal muscle spasm in the lumbar region and neck: two double-blind controlled clinical and laboratory studies," *Archives of Physical Medicine and Rehabilitation,* vol. 59, Feb., 1978, pp. 58-63.

Bean, R. E., *Helping Your Health with Pointed Pressure Therapy.* West Nyack, Parker Publishing Co., 1980.

Biscoe, T. J., and Fry, J. P., "Some pharmacological studies on the spastic mouse," *British Journal of Pharmacology,* vol. 75, 1982, pp. 23-35.

Bradford, S. G., "Characteristics of soft tissue as indicators of health and disease," in *Osteopathic Medicine,* by J. M. Hoag, W. V. Cole, and S. G. Bradford (editors), New York, McGraw-Hill Book Co., 1969, pp. 375-383.

Brendstrup, P. K., "Morphological and chemical connective tissue changes in fibrositic muscle," *Annals of Rheumatic Diseases,* vol. 16, 1957, p. 438.

Brown, B. R., "Cyclobenzaprine in intractable pain syndromes with muscle spasm," *Journal of the American*

Medical Association, vol. 240, no. 11, Sept., 8, 1978, pp. 1151-1152.

Buckley, C. W., "Fibrositis, lumbago and sciatica," *Practitioner,* vol. 134, 1935, pp. 129-134.

Cailliet, R., *Neck and Arm Pain.* Philadelphia, F. A. Davis Co., 1964.

Cailliet, R., *Low Back Pain Syndrome.* Philadelphia, F. A. Davis Co., 1968.

Cailliet, R., *Soft Tissue Pain and Disability.* Philadelphia, F. A. Davis Co., 1977.

Cannon, W. B., *The Wisdom of the Body.* New York, W. W. Norton and Company, Inc., 1932.

Chan, C., *Finger Acupressure.* New York, Ballentine, 1974.

Cheraskin, E., Ringsdorf, W. M., Medford, F. H., and Hicks, B. S., "The musculoskeletal disease proneness profile," *A.C.A. Journal of Chiropractic,* vol. 14, no. 5, May, 1977, S-41-51.

Chicago National College of Naprapathy, "Naprapathy: 1907-1982," Chicago, 1981.

Chicago National College of Naprapathy, *College catalog of the Chicago National College of Naprapathy,* vol. XXX, no. 1, March, 1982.

Chicago Tribune. "Naprapathy is growing health field," Section 15, Sunday, July 18, 1982.

Chusid, J. G., "Nervous system," in *Current Medical Diagnosis and Treatment,* by M. A. Krupp and M. J. Chatton (editors), Los Altos, Lange Medical Publications, 1976, pp. 553-593.

Collins, D. H., "Fibrositis and infection," *Annals of Rheumatic Diseases,* vol. 2, 1940, pp. 114-126.

Coote, J. H., "Central organization of somatosympathetic reflexes," in *Modern Developments in the Principles and Practice of Chiropractic,* by S. Haldeman (editor), New York, Appleton-Century-Crofts, 1980, pp. 107-108.

DeClue, D., "Naprapathy," *Reader,* vol. 7, no. 27, Friday, April, 1978.

Dencklo, M. B., Bemporad, J. R., and MacKay, M. C., "Tics following methylphenidate administration: a report of 20 cases," *Journal of the American Medical Association,* vol. 235, no. 13, March 29, 1976, pp. 1349-1351.

Dorpat, T. L., and Holmes, T. H., "Mechanisms of skeletal muscle pain and fatigue," *A.M.A. Archives of Neurology and Psychiatry,* vol. 74, Dec., 1955, pp. 528-540.

Duke, P., "Healing the natural way," *Centerpiece: A Magazine about You,* vol. 2, no. 8, Sept., 1981.

Duke, P., "Helping our bodies to heal themselves," *Heartland: A Midwest Journal of Health, Sport, Culture and Change,* bibliographic data not available.

Fleet, T., *The Muscle Technique of Concept-Therapy.* San Antonio, Concept Therapy Institute, 1955.

Fryda-Kaurimsky, Z., and Muller-Fassbender, H., "Tizanidine (DS 103-282) in the treatment of acute paravertebral muscle spasm: a controlled trial of comparing Tizanidine and Diazepam," *International Journal of Medical Research,* vol. 9, 1981, pp. 501-505.

Gitelman, R., "A chiropractic approach to biomechanical disorders of the lumbar spine and pelvis," in *Modern Developments in the Principles and Practice of Chiropractic,* by S. Haldeman (editor), New York, Appleton-Century-Crofts, 1980, pp. 297-330.

Glynn, J. H., "Rheumatic pains: some concepts and hypotheses," *Proceedings of the Royal Society of Medicine,* vol. 64, 1971, p. 354.

Gottlieb, W., "Untie those knotted muscles with calcium and vitamin E," *Prevention.* July, 1980. pp. 148-153.

Gottlieb, W., "Tics, tremors and twitches," *Prevention.* Oct., 1980, pp. 131-136.

Grieve, G. P., *Common Vertebral Joint Problems.* Edinburgh, Churchill, Livingstone, 1981.

Guyton, A. C., *Textbook of Medical Physiology.* Philadelphia, W. B. Saunders, 6th edition, 1981.

Haeger, K., "The treatment of peripheral occlusive arterial disease with a-tocopherol as compared with vasodilator agents and antiprothrombin (Dicumarol)," *Vascular Diseases,* vol. 5, 1968, pp. 199-213.

Haeger, K., "Long-time treatment of intermittent claudication with vitamin E," *The American Journal of Clinical Nutrition,* vol. 27, Oct., 1974, pp. 1179-1181.

Haldeman, S., "The release from abnormal musculoskeletal sensory activity," in *Mental Health and Chiropractic,* by H. S. Schwartz (editor), New Hyde Park, Sessions Publishers, 1973, pp. 120-131.

Haldeman, S., "The neurophysiology of spinal pain syndromes," in *Modern Developments in the Principles and Practice of Chiropractic,* by S. Haldeman (editor), New York, Appleton-Century-Crofts, 1980, pp. 119-141.

Hench, P. S., "Rheumatism and arthritis: review of American and English literature: part II," *Annals of Internal Medicine,* vol. 28, 1948, pp. 309-451.

Hennies, O. L., "A new skeletal muscle relaxant (DS 103-282) compared to diazepam in the treatment of muscle spasm of local origin," *Journal of International Medical Research,* vol. 9, 1981, pp. 62-68.

Homewood, A. E., *The Neurodynamics of the Vertebral Subluxation.* St. Petersburg, Valkyrie Press, Inc., 1977.

Illich, I., *Medical Nemesis.* New York, Pantheon Books, 1976.

Jacobson, E., "Imagination, recollection and abstract thinking involving the speech musculature," *American*

Journal of Physiology, vol. 97, no. 1, April, 1931, pp. 200-209.

Jacobson, E., "Electrophysiology of mental activities," *American Journal of Psychology,* vol. 44, Oct., 1932, pp. 677-694.

Jacobson, E., *You Must Relax.* New York, McGraw-Hill Book Co., 1962.

Jordan, H. H., "Myogelosis: the significance of pathologic conditions of musculature in disorders of posture and locomotion," *Archives of Physical Therapy,* vol. 23, 1942, pp. 36-41.

Jowett, R. L., Fidler, M. W., and Troup, J. D. G., "Histochemical changes in the multifidus in mechanical derangement of the spine," *Orthopedic Clinics of North America,* vol. 6, no. 1, Jan., 1975, pp. 145-161.

Kamimura, M., "Comparison of alpha-tocopherol nicotinate and acetate on skin microcirculation," *The American Journal of Clinical Nutrition,* vol. 27, Oct., 1974, pp. 1110-1116.

Karel, L., "The needle effect in the relief of myofascial pain," *Pain,* vol. 6, 1979, pp. 83-90.

Kelsey, J. L., Pastides, H., and Bisbee, G. E., *Musculoskeletal Disorders: Their Frequency of Occurrence and their Impact on the Population of the United States.* New York, Prodist, 1978.

Kennedy, J. L., "Naprapathy—a little-known medical career field," *Chicago Sun-Times.* Wednesday, Sept. 23, 1981.

Kessler, R. M., and Hertling, D., *Management of Common Musculoskeletal Disorders: Physical Therapy Principles and Methods.* Philadelphia, J. B. Lippincott Co., 1983.

Knutsson, E., "Antispastic medication," *Scandinavian Journal of Rehabilitation Medicine,* supplement no. 7, 1980, pp. 80-84.

Korr, I. M., Thomas, P. E., and Wright, H. M., "Symposium on the functional implications of segmental facilitation," *Journal of the American Osteopathic Association,* vol. 54, no. 5, Jan., 1955, pp. 265-282.

Kraft, G. H., Johnson E. W., and LaBan, M. M., "The fibrositis syndrome," *Archives of Physical Medicine and Rehabilitation.* March, 1968, pp. 155-162.

Kruger, H., *Other Healers, Other Cures: A Guide to Alternative Medicine.* Indianapolis, The Bobbs-Merrill Co., Inc., 1974.

Kurland, H. D., *Back Pain: Quick Relief without Drugs.* New York, Simon and Schuster, 1981.

Lehmann, J. F., *Therapeutic Heat and Cold,* Baltimore, Williams and Wilkins, 3rd edition, 1982.

Levine, M., "Chiropractic analysis," in *Mental Health and Chiropractic,* by Schwartz, H. S. (editor), 1973, pp. 81-93.

Levine, J. D., Gromley J., and Fields, H. L., "Observations on the analgesic effects of needle puncture (acupuncture)," *Pain,* vol. 2, 1976, pp. 149-159.

Lowe, J. C., "Calcium and magnesium deficiencies and the vertebral subluxation," *A.C.A. Journal of Chiropractic,* vol. IX, Oct., 1975, S-128-129.

Lowe, J. C., "The nutritional treatment of arthritic diseases," *A.C.A. Journal of Chiropractic,* vol. XI, Sept., 1977, S-89.

Lowe, J. C., "Arthritis: can nutrition help?" *Healthways Magazine,* vol. 32, no. 4, Nov.-Dec., 1977, pp. 6-10.

Lowe, J. C., "The original contingencies hypothesis," *Digest of Chiropractic Economics,* vol. 21, no. 4, Jan-Feb., 1979, pp. 38-113.

Lowe, J. C., "Toxemia," *Texas Chiropractic College Review.* Feb., 1979, pp. 12-13.

Lowe, J. C., "Pangamic acid (vitamin B15) and joint instability due to ligamentous laxity," *Digest of Chiropractic Economics.* July-Aug., 1979, pp. 52-57.

Lowe, J. C., "The nutritional management of muscular dystrophy," *Digest of Chiropractic Economics.* March-April, 1979, pp. 20-135.

Lowe, J. C., "Arthritis of intestinal origin: its correction through diet," *Digest of Chiropractic Economics,* vol. 21, no. 6, May-June, 1979, pp. 14-113.

Lowe, J. C., "The history of man's diet," *Texas Chiropractic College Review.* May, 1979, pp. 22-24.

Lowe, J. C., "Nutrition, ligaments, and the need for spinal manipulation," *Texas Chiropractic College Review.* August, 1979, pp. 25-27.

Lowe, J. C., "Are straight chiropractors covering up a symptom of improper nutrition," *Digest of Chiropractic Economics.* Sept.-Oct., 1979, pp. 56-59.

Lowe, J. C., "Diet, nutrition, and the starting point of chiropractic care," *Today's Chiropractic.* Nov., 1979, pp. 17-20.

Lowe, J. C., "Does high protein intake lead to intestinal toxemia?" *Texas Chiropractic College Review,* vol. 5, no. 4, Nov., 1979, pp. 20-22.

Lowe, J. C., "Improper nutrition: today's foundation of biomechanical stress," *Digest of Chiropractic Economics.* March-April, 1980, pp. 32-35.

Lowe, J. C., "Calcium, magnesium and muscle spasms," *The Chiropractic Family Physician,* vol. 3, no. 6, Sept., 1981, pp. 18-21.

Lowen, A., "The diagnosis of personality from the body," in *Mental Health and Chiropractic,* by H. S. Schwartz (editor), 1973, pp. 53-65.

Lumdervold, A., "Occupational myalgia: electromyographic investigation," *Acta Psychiatry and Neurology,* vol. 26, 1951, pp. 359-369.

Luttges, M. W., and Gerren, R. A., "Compression physiology: nerves and roots," in *Modern Developments in the Principles and Practice of Chiropractic,* by S. Haldeman (editor), New York, Appleton-Century-Crofts, 1980, pp. 65-92.

Mankin, H. J., and Adams, R. D., "Pain in the back and neck," in *Harrison's Principles of Internal Medicine,* by G. W. Thorn, R. A. Adams, E. Braunwald, K. J. Isselbacher, R. G. Petersdorf (editors), New York, McGraw-Hill Book Co., 1977, p. 43.

McDowell, F. H., "Treatment of spasticity," *Drugs,* vol. 22, 1981, pp. 401-408.

Melzack, R., Stillwell, D. M., and Fox, E. J., "Trigger points and acupuncture points for pain: correlations and implications," *Pain,* vol. 3, 1977, pp. 3-23.

Mendelsohn, R. S., *Confessions of a Medical Heretic.* Chicago, Contemporary Books, 1979.

Mendelsohn, R. S., *Male Practice: How Doctors Manipulate Women.* Chicago, Contemporary Books, Inc., 1981.

Moss, R. F., "The curse of the aching back," *Cosmopolitan.* Jan., 1983, pp. 214-218.

Olson, R. E., "Creatine kinase and myofibrillar proteins in hereditary muscular dystrophy and vitamin E deficiency," *The American Journal of Clinical Nutrition,* vol. 27, Oct., 1974, pp. 1117-1129.

Prudden, B., *Pain Erasure: The Bonney Prudden Way.* New York, Ballentine Books, 1980.

Parker Chiropractic Research Foundation, "How well educated is your chiropractor?" form no. 253, 1976.

Pedersen, E., "Management of spasticity on neurophysiological basis," *Scandinavian Journal of Rehabilitation Medicine,* supplement no. 7, 1980, pp. 68-79.

Pelletier, K., *Mind as Healer, Mind as Slayer.* New York, Delta, 1977, p. 65.

Peterson, L., "Denial of educational opportunities—an educational puzzle," *Palmer Chiropractic College Alumni News,* vol. XXII, no. 3, July, 1982, pp. 11-12.

Plutchik, R., "The role of muscular tension in maladjustment," *The Journal of General Psychology,* vol. 50, 1954, pp. 45-62.

Report of the Select Committee on Nutrition and Human Needs, U. S. Senate. Forward by Senator George McGovern. *Eating in America: Dietary Goals for the United States.* Cambridge, MIT Press, Jan. 14, 1977.

Sato, A., "Physiological studies of the somatoautonomic reflexes," in *Modern Developments in the Principles and Practice of Chiropractic,* by S. Haldeman (editor), New York, Appleton-Century-Crofts, 1980, pp. 93-105.

Schier, M. J., "Muscle cramp pain may indicate more serious disorder, doctor says," *Houston Post.* Friday, March 11, 1983.

Schubert, M., and Hamerman, D., *A Primer on Connective Tissue Biochemistry.* Philadelphia, Lea and Febiger, 1968.

Schwartz, H. S., "The psychotherapeutic experience of chiropractic," in *Mental Health and Chiropractic,* by H. S. Schwartz (editor), 1973, pp. 161-173.

Schwartz, H. S., and Moulton, D., "Integrated therapeutic procedure within the framework of comprehensive chiropractic," in *Mental Health and Chiropractic,* by H. S. Schwartz (editor), 1973, pp. 195-215.

Scott, D. S., "Myofascial pain—dysfunction syndrome: a psychobiological perspective," *Journal of Behavioral Medicine,* vol. 4, no. 4, 1981, pp. 451-465.

Selye, H., *The Stress of Life.* New York, McGraw-Hill Book Co., 1956.

Shaw, L., "The spasm theory of heart attack," *Prevention.* Oct., 1979, pp. 106-110.

Shepherd, W. D., "Subclavian muscle spasm and headache," *Digest of Chiropractic Economics.* July-August, 1982, pp. 46-47.

Shestack, R., *Handbook of Physical Therapy.* New York, Springer Publishing Co., 3rd edition, 1977.

Simons, D. G., "Muscle pain syndromes—part I," *American Journal of Physical Medicine,* vol. 54, no. 6, 1975, pp. 289-311.

Simons, D. G., "Muscle pain syndromes—part II," *American Journal of Physical Medicine,* vol. 55, no. 1, 1976, pp. 15-42.

Slocumb, C. H., "Fibrositis," *Clinics,* vol. 2, 1943, pp. 169-178.

Sola, A. E., and Williams R. L., "Myofascial pain syndromes," *Neurology,* vol. VI, Jan.-Dec., 1956, pp. 91-95.

Stein, M., "Influence of brain and behavior on the immune system," *Science,* vol. 166, 1969, pp. 435-440.

Steindler, A., and Luck, J. V., "Differential diagnosis of pain low in the back," *Journal of the American Medical Association,* vol. 110, no. 2, Jan. 8, 1938.

Stenger, R. J., Spiro, D., Schully, R. E., and Shannon, J. M., "Ultrastructural and physiologic alterations in ischemic skeletal muscle," *American Journal of Pathology,* vol. 40, 1962, pp. 1-20.

Suh, C. H., "Computer-aided spinal biomechanics," in *Modern Developments in the Principles and Practice of Chiropractic,* by S. Haldeman (editor), New York, Appleton-Century-Crofts, 1980, pp. 143-170.

Sunderland, S., "The anatomy of the intervertebral foramen and the mechanisms of compression and stretch of nerve roots," in *Modern Developments in the Principles and Practice of Chiropractic,* by S. Haldeman (editor), New York, Appleton-Century-Crofts, 1980, pp. 45-64.

Thach, B. T., Chase, T. N., and Bosma, J. F., "Oral facial dyskinesia associated with prolonged use of antihistaminic decongestants," *Lancet.* vol. 293, no. 10, 1969, pp. 1388-1390.

Travell, J., Rinzler, S., and Herman M., "Pain and disability of the shoulder and arm," *Journal of the American Medical Association,* vol. 120, no. 6, Oct. 10, 1942, pp. 417-422.

Travell, J., "Rapid relief of acute 'stiff neck' by ethyl chloride spray," *American Medical Women's Association,* vol. 4, no. 3, March, 1949, pp. 89-95.

Travell, J., "Ethyl chloride spray for painful muscle spasm," *Archives of Physical Medicine,* vol. XXXIII, no. 1, May, 1952, pp. 291-298.

Travell, J., and Simons, D. G., *Myofascial Pain and Dysfunction: The Trigger Point Manual.* Baltimore, Williams and Wilkins, 1983.

Vannerson, J. F., "Some comments on the weak muscle theory," *Digest of Chiropractic Economics,* vol. 25, no. 2, Sept.-Oct., 1982, pp. 52-148.

Wilk, C. A., *Chiropractic Speaks Out: A Reply to Medical Propaganda, Bigotry, and Ignorance.* Park Ridge, Wilk Publishing Co., 1973.

Williams, R. J., *Biochemical Individuality.* Austin, University of Texas Press, 1956.

Yarom, R., and Robin, G. C., "Studies on spinal and peripheral muscles from patients with scoliosis," *Spine,* vol. 4, no. 1, Jan.-Feb., 1979, pp. 12-21.

Young, R. R., Rebeiz, J., and Adams, R. D., "Diseases of striated muscle," in *Harrison's Principles of Internal Medicine,* by G. W. Thorn, R. A. Adams, E. Braunwald, K. J. Isselbacher, R. G. Petersdorf (editors), New York, McGraw-Hill Book Co., 1977, p. 1972.

Spasm

Young, R. R., and Delwaide, P. J., "Drug therapy: spasticity," *The New England Journal of Medicine,* vol. 304, no. 1, Jan. 1, 1981, pp. 28-33.

Young, R. R., and Delwaide, P. J., "Drug therapy: spasticity," *The New England Journal of Medicine,* vol. 304, no. 2, Jan. 8, 1981, pp. 96-99.

INDEX